March 31, 2006

To Phyllis
Gaster
with fondness

More Grace Than Glamour

This book made possible by:

Bank of Oklahoma, N.A.
Henry Browne
Jim C. Clark
Frank & Judy Elmore
Ed & Barbara Eskridge
Eloise Gamble
Gerald L. Gamble
Jim & Mary Newby Gamble
David & Barbara Green
Michael & Madeline Gulotta
Kirk & Dana Humphreys
Helene Jayroe
Frank & Cathy Keating
Kerr-McGee Corporation
Kurt & Cathy Leichter
Herman & LaDonna Meinders
George & Anna Arganbright Milleret
The Norick Family
Oklahoma City University
Duard & Anne Pyle
Tom & Bobbie Roe
Adair & Peggy Smith
Skip & Mary Mitchell Trimble

More Grace Than Glamour

My Life as Miss America and Beyond

Jane Jayroe with Bob Burke

Foreword by Jimmy Webb

OKLAHOMA VOICES SERIES

SERIES EDITOR: GINI MOORE CAMPBELL

ASSOCIATE EDITOR: ERIC DABNEY

Printed in the United States of America.
ISBN 1-885596-52-9
Library of Congress Catalog Number 2005938933
Designed by Carol Haralson

Unless otherwise noted, photographs are courtesy
of Jane Jayroe Gamble.

OKLAHOMA HERITAGE ASSOCIATION

DEDICATED TO MY MOTHER,
HELENE GRACE JAYROE, ANOTHER AMAZING GRACE,
AND HER LOVING LEGACY:

TYLER, ELAINE, LUKE MICHAEL, AND MAYA KATHRYN;
JACE, CECE, HANNAH ELIZABETH,
DITA GRACE, AND DAXX JAYROE;
DAL, CARIE, JAYDEN CASE, KESS ADAIR, AND
AVA GRACE ; CADE AND JACQUI

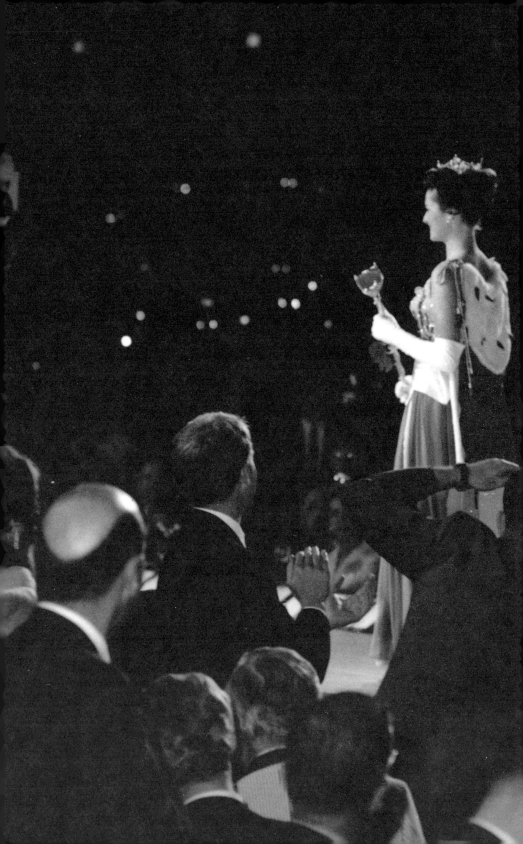

Contents

Gratitudes

To my mother, Helene Jayroe, whose mind and memory provide the information for much of the book. Without her organizational skills, I would not have one scrapbook. She found details that were lost to me forever. She is forever and always my momma, my grace, and my blessing.

To my sister, Judy, who is always supportive in any effort. She helped with pictures and last minute details. Her mind is as cluttered as mine, so we have forgotten a lot of our joint history, but we have fun remembering what we can. Having a sister like Judy is the best.

To my husband, Jerry, who survived the many trips down my memory lane while writing this book. Also thanks for his tolerance of my growing pile of stuff that covered the library and then the hall and then finally took over the dining room. His support and love are everything to me.

To my friend, Connie Thrash McGoodwin, who was willing to listen to me go over so many memories and help me sort through my life. Thanks to Connie for reading the book and providing the balanced perspective that she is so good at doing.

To my friend, Sue Hale—Sister Sue I call her—and Linda Lynn, Melissa Hayer, Mary Phillips, Robin Davison, and Billie Harry at the Oklahoma Publishing Company who helped gather and select photographs.

To Norman Neaves, Trevor Hudson, and Church of the Servant for the spiritual support that encourages me to "tell the whole truth" about my life in the hope that the dark spots will lead someone else to the light.

To my new best friend, Bob Burke. I am forever in the debt of this great writer and greater human being for this project. It was pure joy to work on the book because of his organizational skills, outstanding writing ability,

9

incredibly fun personality, and deep spirit of joy. More than anything I appreciate his interest in my life and constant encouragement that said "Yes, someone will be interested in this." Thanks to George and Marcia Davis, Hayley Miller, John Millar, Lisa Angelotti, Erin Kistler, Blake Hamilton, Kathy Morley, Leah Kayajanian, Sarah Farris, Ryan Baker, Peter Zhmutski, and Elvin Richmond for proofreading the manuscript, and to Debbie Neill, Amy Clakley, and Katherine Schmidt for editorial assistance. I appreciate the assistance of our editors, Gini Moore Campbell and Eric Dabney, and Carol Haralson for agreeing to lend her incredible talent to the book's design. ~ JANE JAYROE GAMBLE, 2005

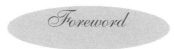

Foreword

MY RELATIONSHIP with music began early in life. My father was a preacher and my mother's lifelong dream was for me to be the piano player of the church. When I was about six years old, she began an intensive effort to make me a pianist. If I missed practices, she took away privileges. She was the driving force behind what became a passion for the keyboard.

By the time I was 12, I was playing fulltime for church services. However, there was something inside me that wanted to add to the notes written in the church hymnal. Heavily influenced by the more folkoriented hymns from Ireland, Scotland, and England such as "I Will Arise," "Come Thy Fount," and "Amazing Grace," I began slipping into my own minor-chord arrangements, much to the consternation of my father and some members of the congregation.

The melodies from the church hymns blended with country, folk, and pop tunes that I heard. Soon, I began writing my own songs. I discovered that the great joy of my craft is to take me on a lifelong voyage across many distant and wondrous musical seas.

I was, and still am, a romanticist. I wanted to capture and involve the emotions of anyone listening to my songs. I liked words—the way they clash around together and bang up against each other, especially in songs. I spent hours at the piano dreaming of new combinations of notes and words to accompany them.

At Laverne High School I met Jane Jayroe. She was an incredible singer and loved my music. Even more valuable was her kindness to me. Jane became my best friend. It was not uncommon for her to sit on the piano bench with me and sing the words of some new song I had just written. Her pleasant vocals gave life to some of my earliest compositions.

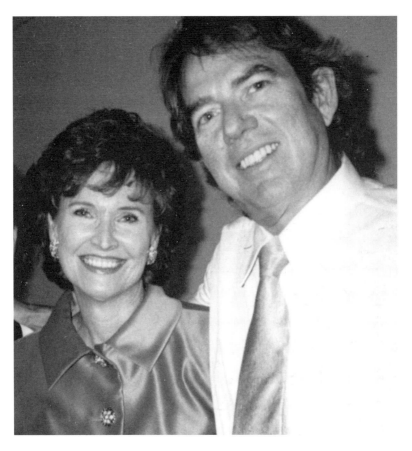

Jimmy Webb and I visit on one of his frequent trips back to Oklahoma.
We have been friends since high school.

Some of the highlights of my high school years came when Jane asked me to write the lyrics and music for songs for special programs in which she was singing. It was a special feeling when all the people of our little town gathered in the high school auditorium to hear Jane sing and me play the piano. We even traveled to Oklahoma City to audition for a locally famous television show. We didn't make it—but you'll have to read this book to find out why!

I have never forgotten my Oklahoma roots. I have been honored to be asked to appear at Oklahoma's celebrations, to write music for the U.S. Olympic Festival and other events. Tears came to my eyes the night we dedicated the new dome on the State Capitol. I loved to see a Native American on the top of the dome. My great grandmother was Cherokee and my emotions got the best of me.

My Oklahoma roots have provided me at least three great pleasures in life—my induction into the Oklahoma Hall of Fame, being asked to write the official song for the celebration of Oklahoma's Centennial, and my decades-long friendship with Jane. Whether we visit at huge celebrations or in the privacy of dinner, we easily revert back to the 1960s when an aspiring young singer and her friend, a piano playing teenager, made great music together—not knowing what lay ahead in their lives. — JIMMY WEBB, 2005

Jimmy Webb's songs carry an inimitable signature of strong rhythm, inventive musical structure, and rich harmonies—all wrapped in emotion and sometimes romance. He was the first artist in history to receive Grammy awards for music, lyrics, and orchestration. Jimmy is best known for instant classics he provided for such artists as Glen Campbell—"By the Time I Get to Phoenix" and "Wichita Lineman"; for Richard Harris—"MacArthur Park" and "Didn't We"; for the Fifth Dimension—"Up, Up and Away"; and for Joe Cocker—"The Moon's a Harsh Mistress." Linda Ronstadt said Jimmy's songs "have 17-layer emotions and sophisticated chord changes that are absolutely dazzling." Frank Sinatra called "By the Time I Get to Phoenix" the greatest torch song ever written. Jimmy's friend, Michael Feinstein, says Jimmy is a master of this musical era.

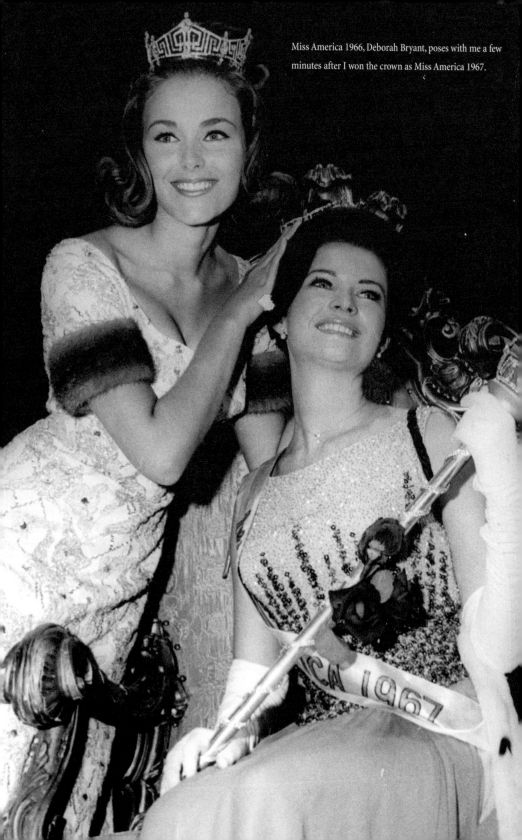

Miss America 1966, Deborah Bryant, poses with me a few minutes after I won the crown as Miss America 1967.

1

Prologue

I t was a moment like no other—a moment of which most little girls growing up in America dream. I was standing on the end of a runway in Atlantic City, New Jersey. I had a crown on my head and Bert Parks was singing, "There she is, Miss America!" He was singing to me! Memories of all the Miss America pageants I had watched since childhood came rushing back to my mind. Bert Parks was singing to me! I was Miss America!

"Don't cry!" I kept telling myself. Crying for some people meant dainty tears that add a little shine and an image of sincerity for their face. But for Jane Anne Jayroe, crying was not pretty. Crying for me was far from tears cascading down my cheek—it was swollen red eyes, running mascara, a drippy nose, and a blotchy face. I knew that if I lost control of the moment, floods of tears would gush from my eyes and embarrass all those who had worked so hard to get me to this moment in history.

A tidal wave of emotions engulfed my very soul. The crowd was on its feet cheering. The jam-packed auditorium was ablaze with lights. I was blinded by flashes from what seemed like a thousand cameras.

I could not believe what was happening. I was a 19-year-old shy, unsophisticated college girl from Laverne, Oklahoma, a town of less than 2,000 people, and had just received what was at the time one of the most recognizable titles in the world.

I was scared to death. I was like a little girl who would run outside to sing and dance in the glitter of God's sunshine. I had dreamed of dashing over the hill, but at the first sign of a raindrop, rushing back into the house to hide behind my mother's legs and hold onto something I could see and feel and trust. I would peek out to see if the world was safe for my dreams and fantasies.

But there was no hiding from this very public moment. What a whirlwind week it had been. It was an unbelievable experience to go from being a girl from Laverne who played high school basketball and who had never flown in an airplane to being catapulted into the center of a nation's attention.

I had not expected to win. Sure, I had practiced for years walking in a bathing suit, singing, and performing. I was the reigning Miss Oklahoma, but surely there were dozens of other girls who more deserved to be called "Miss America."

It was not that I did not want to win the contest. I loved competition. But throughout the week, I expected Miss America to be someone like Miss California, Charlene Diane Dallas. She traveled with an entourage of hairdressers and coaches and her evening gown cost $1,000, a fortune in 1966. I was in Atlantic City with my sweet family and almost no one else, not even the Miss Oklahoma pageant director. Charlene was the girl I thought would walk the runway with a huge bouquet of roses and the Miss America sash. She was Hollywood beautiful and San Francisco sophisticated.

I would have been perfectly happy to finish in the top ten. I really was not even nervous when Charlene and I were the only two girls left standing on the enormous stage under the bright lights. I knew that everyone in my hometown was sitting in front of a television set. Many of my neighbors in Laverne had gathered at my parents' house to watch their new color set. I also knew that my friends at Oklahoma City University were hovered around their televisions.

I had made the top two—I had won everything I wanted. Being first runner up to Miss America was an incredible honor, so I did not worry for a second about the final announcement, especially when I saw the paper in Bert Parks' hand as he walked from the judges' table to stand beside us. He had inadvertently turned the paper so I could see the words "Miss California." What I did not know was that the judges had written down the name of the first runner up.

When Miss California was announced as first runner up, I was so stunned I could hardly breathe. It had to be a mistake! I was not supposed to win! I wanted to drive home with my parents, go to college, see my boyfriend, drive the Miss Oklahoma car, and be with my friends. This could not be happening.

The reality of the moment and memories of my childhood clouded my thought process. I had been dreaming about this runway and the joy of competing my entire life, but when it got right down to the basics, I was too afraid of being Miss America to be "her" in 1966.

A dream is one thing—this was real. For a moment, I did not even trust God with this big job, to make me into something that I surely was not—Miss America! With flash bulbs still popping, I ascended my throne as the winner of the world's greatest beauty pageant. Along the way, I stepped on my dress and tore a hole in it—typical me—no royalty here!

Even though I appeared to be in control of my emotions, I was not. The whole world, or at least the millions of people watching on television, surely recognized my state of mind when Bert Parks asked me how I felt, and I blubbered with emotion, "Without my parents, I wouldn't be here!" Nothing like me stating the obvious.

Finally, the endless moment was over. I wanted to talk to my mother and father and have some time to think, but the worst was yet to come. I was literally captured on the stage by an army of photographers. Then came the real shock—I was escorted out of Convention Hall by police officers. My family was lost in the throng of people who charged toward me, yelling, wanting to touch my gown, scaring me to death. I kept thinking, "What next?"

I had no idea what the next year had in store for me. I would learn to depend upon grace—not the kind of grace that a beauty queen displays when she walks a runway, but the grace of God. I would learn that God's grace is not deserved, but free to all who ask. More than once I would lean upon a scripture verse found in II Corinthians 12:9, "God's grace is sufficient for us for His power is made perfect in weakness." I like Dallas Willard's definition of grace as the action of God bringing to pass in our lives good things that we neither deserve nor are capable of accomplishing on our own.

That grace is the "grace" of my story.

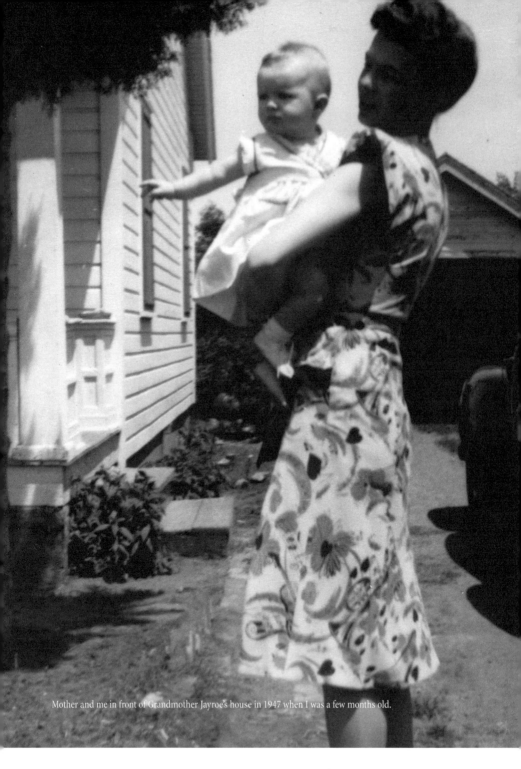

Mother and me in front of Grandmother Jayroe's house in 1947 when I was a few months old.

2

A BLESSED HERITAGE

*W*ithout a doubt, God's greatest blessing in my life was having Pete and Helene Jayroe as parents and Judy as my sister. I cannot imagine life without them.

Daddy's name was E.G. Jayroe, born June 4, 1919, in Sentinel, in Washita County, Oklahoma. Given the nickname, "Pete" early in life, he was one of five sons of William T. and Lettie A. McKee Jayroe, a hearty farm couple who tilled the soil and loved the land on which they lived. Two of their boys, Price and Chester, died early in life.

Washita County, in the heart of west-central Oklahoma, is named for the Washita River that flows through the county. Sentinel, the southwestern part of Washita County, was named for a newspaper published at nearby Cloud Chief. The post office at Sentinel was established March 6, 1899.

Daddy and his family farmed the red land around Sentinel during the Great Depression, the worst and longest period of high unemployment and low business activity in modern history. The Depression had a mighty grip on Oklahoma during the 1930s. It began in 1929 with the crash of the stock market and worsened as banks failed, farms were auctioned to pay mortgages, factories closed, and millions of Americans were left homeless and jobless.

As if the crippled economy was not enough, western Oklahoma was plagued with dust storms that blew away thousands of acres of precious top soil. Sand blew in such quantities that chickens went to roost at noon, travelers lost their way, airports closed, and trains stopped.

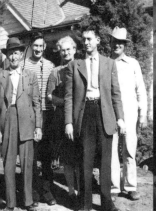

Daddy's family—left to right, W.T. Jayroe, Daddy, Lettie Jayroe, Bill Jayroe, and Sam Jayroe.

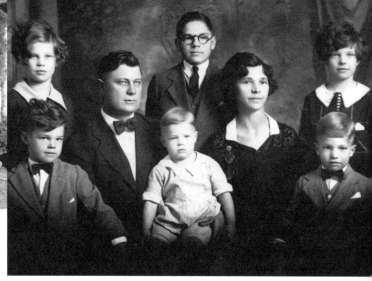

My mother's family in 1928. Children in front, left to right, H.L. Smith, Adair Smith, and Maynard Smith. In back, Honore Smith, Homer Lyle Smith, Boyd Smith, Clara May Smith, and Helene Smith.

Somehow, my grandparents held onto their land and grew enough crops to feed their family and animals. My grandfather Jayroe worked from sunup to sundown on his land, although after the deaths of his two sons, some say he gave up on life. He loved to spend time playing dominos in the pool hall. I remember going in and asking him for a nickel or dime. He would have given me anything, but I soon got the word that little girls were not supposed to be in the pool hall.

My stalwart grandmother was a hardy and stout woman who could wring the neck from a chicken with the quickest snap and outwork many men in the arena of manual farm labor. She loved everything about farming. When in her later years she was confined to a nursing home, her great joy was to ride in a car and look at growing crops and freshly plowed fields.

My mother, Helene Grace Smith Jayroe, was born February 16, 1919, in Turpin, Oklahoma. The town, originally called Lorena, and located in northwestern Beaver County in the Oklahoma Panhandle, was named for Oklahoma City railroad developer C.J. Turpin in 1925.

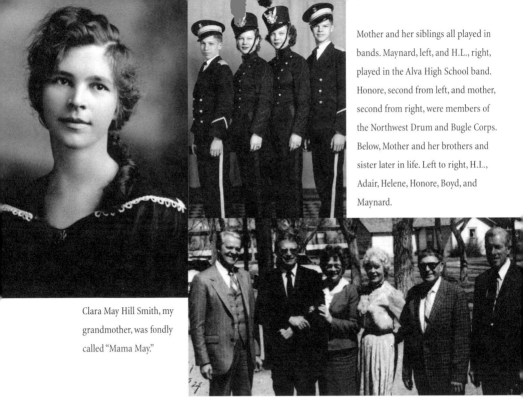

Mother and her siblings all played in bands. Maynard, left, and H.L., right, played in the Alva High School band. Honore, second from left, and mother, second from right, were members of the Northwest Drum and Bugle Corps. Below, Mother and her brothers and sister later in life. Left to right, H.L., Adair, Helene, Honore, Boyd, and Maynard.

Clara May Hill Smith, my grandmother, was fondly called "Mama May."

My maternal grandmother, Clara May Hill Smith, was born in 1884 in Illinois and came with her family to homestead land in the Panhandle. My great grandfather, George Hill, was one of the early pioneers of the Panhandle that became known as No Man's Land when federal legislation failed to add the land to any existing state. All my grandparents came to Oklahoma from eastern states, looking for a dream and an opportunity to create their own future. They were hearty, courageous, tough, and believed strongly in God's guidance in their lives. My Grandparents Hill helped start the First Methodist Church in Turpin and taught Sunday school and sang in the choir.

Grandmother's brother, Boyd Almon Hill, introduced football at Oklahoma A & M College, now Oklahoma State University, in Stillwater. A former student at West Point, Hill led the A & M football team in 1906.

Grandmother Smith was fondly called "Mama May" by her grandchildren. She married Homer Lyle Smith, a wonderful man we called "Oklahoma Dad." My mother, like my father, was born into a hardworking farm family. She was one of six children, a lot of mouths to feed during the hard years of the Great Depression. Oklahoma Dad often worked more than one job to keep his family in food and clothing.

Music was king in Mama May's home. Oklahoma Dad was an accomplished musician and all the children played instruments. Saturday nights were special in the Smith home. Following a huge country meal prepared by Mama May, Oklahoma Dad and his children removed their instruments from under the bed and off the walls and played until bedtime.

After living in Kansas for awhile, Oklahoma Dad and Mama May moved back to Turpin in 1931. These were hard days during the Great Depression. Oklahoma Dad lost at least two of his farms. The others he farmed for other landowners. He lost money in the bank and his home in Liberal, Kansas. And yet mother never remembered being deprived. Everyone was in the same boat and helped each other. She always told me, "It wasn't hard to go without."

Oklahoma Dad and Mama May were disappointed that the hard times caused many of their friends to leave Oklahoma. On a Sunday in 1931, the rent house in which the Smiths were living burned to the ground. It was a blessing that the family was not at home because there was an explosion and the house was completely destroyed. Neighbors gave my grandparents whatever they needed from their meager supplies. One lady took my mother home after school and made her five dresses out of feed sack cloth.

In 1934, the family moved to Alva where there was a better opportunity for college. Higher education was a big deal to Homer and May Smith. Oklahoma Dad drove from Alva to Turpin to farm, but the family planted themselves where the children would have the greatest opportunity to attend college. All six of the Smith children eventually received a college degree, and many of them earned advanced degrees, quite an accomplishment for an Oklahoma farm family in the first half of the 20th century.

When I was young, Mama May recited the stories of her early life, hard times of prairie fires, coyotes stealing watermelon crops, and trying to serve meals during the dust bowl days. Mama May was the first school teacher in the Independence school district and a lifelong member of the Women's Christian Temperance Union. As a pioneer teacher, she earned only $10 a month.

My mother graduated from high school in Alva in 1936. Four years later, on July 23, 1940, she married my daddy in Medicine Lodge, Kansas. They had met at Northwestern State College at Alva where daddy was on a basketball scholarship. He had played basketball for a short time for the legendary Henry Iba at Oklahoma A & M, but transferred to the smaller college at Alva after his first year. Being from a small town, daddy had a tough time adjusting to the campus life at Oklahoma A & M.

Mother has always said that it made no sense for her and daddy to get married. They had no money and no plans for any money. However, it was a wonderful marriage that endured until daddy's death.

Mother and daddy, below right, were married July 23, 1940, at Medicine Lodge, Kansas. The photograph below left was taken a month later with mother's family. Left to right, John Mitchell, Honore Smith, Mama May, Oklahoma Dad, mother, and daddy. Daddy was a very good high school and college basketball player.

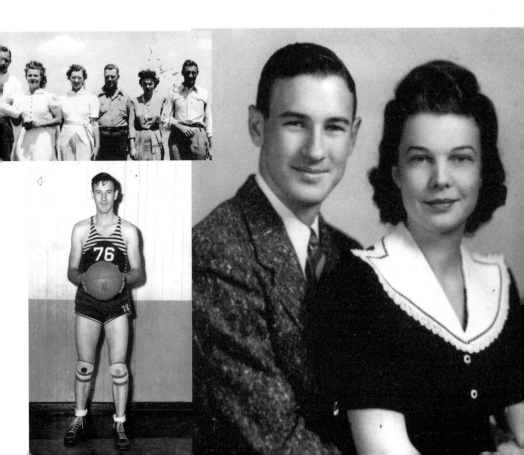

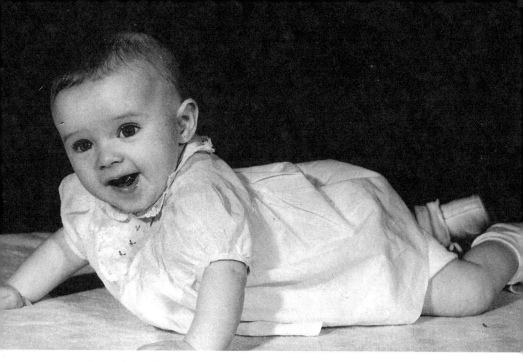

I was born in Clinton, Oklahoma, as the second daughter to Pete and Helene Jayroe.

In 1942, daddy transferred to Southwestern State Teachers College in Weatherford, Oklahoma, where he played for Coach Rankin Williams. Among daddy's teammates was Abe Lemons, the future basketball coach at Oklahoma City University and the University of Texas. They were fast friends. When I became Miss America, Abe wrote daddy a note saying to come see him when he was in Oklahoma City because he had been practicing his "curtsy." Abe was a priceless treasure!

While daddy was completing college, mother gave birth to my sister, Judith May "Judy" Jayroe, on March 30, 1942, in Weatherford. Judy was the first grandchild on my mother's side of the family, a very special event. Mother graduated from Southwestern and taught school at Elk City in 1943 and 1944.

After Daddy graduated from college, he joined the United States Navy. The fighting of World War II was hot and heavy and daddy believed he owed his country service in the military. In 1944, mother and Judy followed him to San Diego, California. They returned to Hammon, Oklahoma, in 1946 where daddy coached some great teams.

I was born in nearby Clinton, Oklahoma on October 30, 1946. My mother's doctor was Curtis Cunningham. When I was born, Dr. Cunningham told mother I was such a pretty baby. Then he placed a finger on her nose and said, "All of my babies are pretty." We moved to Sentinel in 1949.

My childhood seemed perfect. My older sister, who had helped name me, was like a second mother. My parents had lots of friends and they enjoyed life. In fact, they loved life, they loved basketball, they loved students at the school where they taught, and they loved their family.

My sister and I never doubted the devotion we felt from our parents. Basketball was a great part of our life because daddy was a basketball coach in his hometown for Sentinel High School. In Sentinel, we lived across the street from the school where my daddy coached and my mother taught fifth grade.

Family was so important to my childhood. Left to right, my sister, Judy, cousin, Sammie Jayroe, holding me, and cousin, Barbara Jean Jayroe. This photograph was taken in 1947.

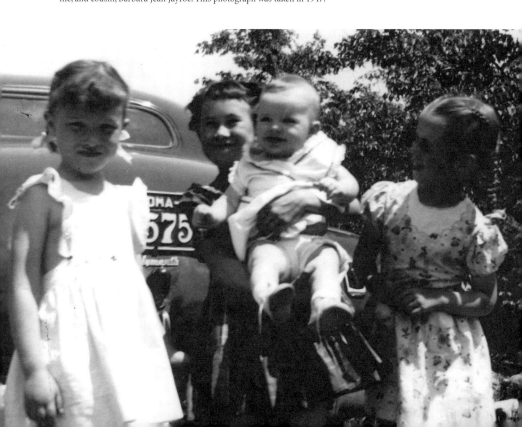

During basketball season, Judy and I sat with mother at the games while daddy coached the team. For road games, we all rode the school bus together. Being the baby of the coach, I was passed around like the mascot of the pep club. I learned early that I should not bother daddy during a game. He was focused. At the end of the game, I asked my mother, "Who winded?" instead of "Who won?" At tournament games, especially the district tournament that was usually held in Cordell, I stayed clear of both mother and daddy. I just played with other children and left them with all the stresses.

When I was very young, Grandfather Jayroe died. It was a sad occasion for our family, but I was fortunate to have more Jayroe family in the area. I enjoyed visiting with my Uncle Sam and Aunt Edith Jayroe, and their daughter, Sammie. She was my only cousin in town and a generous and fun friend. Summers in western Oklahoma were unforgettable. Daddy took whatever summer jobs were available to supplement the low wages being paid Oklahoma teachers in the 1950s. Many summers daddy farmed or worked as an adjuster for an insurance company on crop losses caused by Oklahoma's frequent hailstorms. When he was not working summer jobs, daddy earned his masters degree in administration from the University of Oklahoma.

We loved water sports and working in the yard. My mother had a unique way of making everything fun, whether it was pulling weeds from a flower bed or swimming at Lugert Lake near Altus or at municipal pools in Hobart and Cordell.

I was introduced to racial segregation at the swimming pool in Clinton. I did not understand why African American children were not allowed to swim with us because my family, Mama May in particular, had very strict rules about respecting all people and recognizing that God loved all people of all races the same.

Mama May continued to be a great influence on Judy and me. She and mother both corrected our incorrect grammar, regardless of the colloquialisms of the area in which we lived. Mama May had very high standards for the beauty she created. She enforced her rules for manners and good behavior with such a loving hand that no grandchild ever felt they were unjustly reprimanded.

I remember one incident involving Mama May's rules. She had a towel to dry dishes, a towel for drying hands, and rules about placing only certain items in her waste baskets which she had tediously lined with paper. One morning I blew my nose and placed the tissue in the clean waste basket. Mama May said because of the germs on the tissue, I should have deposited it in the toilet in the restroom. The next day, when I ate a banana, I thought, "Maybe the banana has germs too, so I should put the banana peel in the stool." I quickly learned what problems that could cause.

Even though daddy's coaching job was the primary focus of my young life, mother, Judy, and I were very active in the First Methodist Church. Later, through mother's influence, daddy joined the church and we were baptized one wonderful night by Reverend Gillingham.

Most of my friends in my early life were associated with church. There were no children my age in our neighborhood so I longed for time with my friends at Sunday school and latter at youth group on Sunday evenings. My mother was a shining example of service in the church. She was active in the education program and spearheaded efforts for the women of the church to serve lunch for the local Rotary Club as a fund raising activity. She was very busy—but her being busy never took her away from the family.

Mother even made service in the church fun for her daughters. On Tuesday nights we went to the grocery store and bought food for the Rotary Club luncheon on Wednesdays. She taught school all morning, and rushed to the church to help other volunteer cooks serve the Rotarians. I helped also. My sister was either involved in the music for the program or helped serve. What a wonderful legacy of service mother left to all of us. She taught me the great value of volunteering in your community.

A remarkable advantage to growing up in a small town in the 1950s was the amount of freedom children had. We roamed all over town, looking for interesting things to do. Safety was not an issue. Later, I rode my bicycle all over town, and my parents never feared for my safety.

Most of my same-age classmates lived on farms outside Sentinel so my parents would often let me go home with them after Sunday church. With only a few friends in town, I spent a great deal of my early years playing alone. I had a vivid imagination and remember sitting in a tree in our front yard creating entire stories. I presided over burials of many dead birds. I played Pocahontas on the streets of Sentinel.

Our family loved animals—dogs, cats, and especially horses. We had a Cocker Spaniel named Pedro and our favorite dog, an English Boston Bulldog named Phoebe. Daddy bought me what we thought was a gentle horse. But, the animal had apparently been drugged during the sale and was in fact a difficult pony that went wild when she was saddled. The horse—I named her Lady—had a problem with a leg so mother and I rubbed down the leg twice a day the first summer we had her. Eventually, I was able to ride Lady bareback, although daddy had to sell her because she continually tried to throw me off.

My parents taught Judy and me that hard work was good for the soul. We were expected to pick cotton every fall as the fluffy bolls matured. Judy was excited about pulling bolls during the two weeks that school recessed during cotton picking season because it enabled her to save enough money to buy new school clothes. I was less excited because I did not care about having new clothing. However, one year I happily consented to go to the fields with Judy in return for getting a new puppy at the end of the cotton harvest.

Growing up in rural Oklahoma gave me a keen appreciation for the different seasons of the year and their special scents. One of my fondest memories was of picking cotton during an Indian summer day when the shadows from the trees began to creep over the cotton field. The smell of the earth changed during that time of the year. The scent of he earth, the early hint of fall, and the cotton all created a special fall bouquet that I recall with fondness. I knew that it would not be long until the weather would turn cool and the trees would lose their leaves.

The same appreciation for the smell of Oklahoma's changing seasons also came during wheat harvest in the spring. Each year we usually traveled to Turpin where we would help my Grandfather Smith harvest his wheat fields. The earth, when giving up its bounty, has its own aroma, and when mixed with the changing seasons and an occasional spring rain, the scents are spectacular.

Mother helped cook for the men who worked past dark bringing the golden grain from the fields. We would sit around a huge table with my mother's family and laugh way past my normal bed time.

I was so blessed to be surrounded by loving family.

JUDY JAYROE ELMORE

~ ~ ~ *"Janie is a perfect little sister. She was born beautiful and bright, and then grew into an exquisite, intelligent woman. As a little girl, she was a bit shy. She learned early in life to just stand and smile, which made people say, 'What a pretty little girl with such a pretty smile,' instead of, 'My, isn't she shy?' I had to sell her Girl Scout cookies for her because she was too shy to approach anyone. We literally had to 'make' her sing specials at church. Even in the midst of all her successes, she never loses sight of the importance of God, family, and friends. She is humble, honest, giving, sincere, and trustworthy. She is my best friend."*

JUDGE TIM LEONARD

~ ~ ~ *"While Jane has had many accomplishments and great success, both personally and professionally, she has always maintained her values learned from her loving parents and supportive neighbors in her hometown. Growing up and living in a small town close by, I know the pride that the whole community has always felt about her success. She in turn has been proud of her heritage and appreciated the support she has received from all Oklahomans."*

BRUCE DAY

~ ~ ~ *"My long term friendship with Jane has been, in part, based upon our small town western Oklahoma backgrounds. Who, among her many friends, would deny that a great part of the charm of this graceful woman is based on her obvious and truthful goodwill toward her fellow man. Her small town upbringing fostered this trait. She has worn it well."*

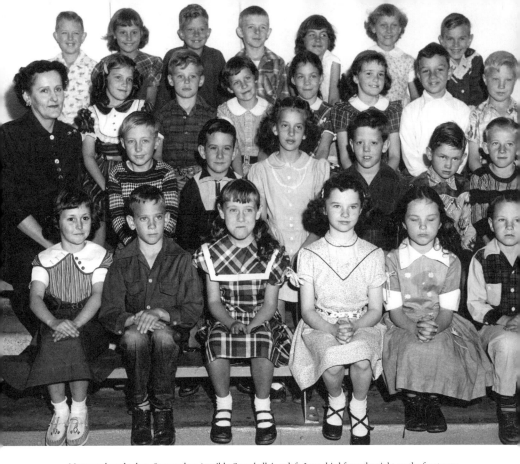

My second grade class. Our teacher, Armilda Campbell, is at left. I am third from the right on the front row.

3

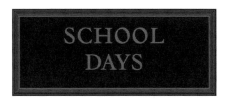

SCHOOL DAYS

$\mathcal{I}$ began my formal education in Sentinel in 1952. My first grade teacher was Miss Blanche Thomas, a dear, sweet woman who had also been my dad's first grade teacher 25 years before. Dan Stowers, the son of a Sentinel physician, was my best friend. I was somewhat of a tomboy and most of my good friends were boys.

Dan and I often fought after school, although we both knew we would remain friends. We had to, because our parents were very close and the families spent a lot of time together. One day in the first grade when school recessed for the day, I splashed through mud puddles and soiled my clothing. A teacher took me to my mother's seventh grade class. I was traumatized when my dirty clothing was removed and I was placed in a seventh-grade boy's jacket. I was very shy and hesitant to tell the student that he could not have his jacket after class because my clothes were being washed and dried.

In the second grade, my best friend was actually a girl, Susie Beard. Also in my class was Gary Lumpkin, the presiding judge of the Oklahoma Court of Criminal Appeals. My grade school teachers, Miss Thomas, Armilda Campbell, Maude Edgar, Susan McCombs, and Thelma Vaughn were wonderful. My fifth grade teacher, of course, was my mother. It was a little strange addressing your teacher as "mother," but the other children did not mind. I think mother gave me lower grades than any other teacher, but she worked overtime trying to show other students she was not partial to her own daughter.

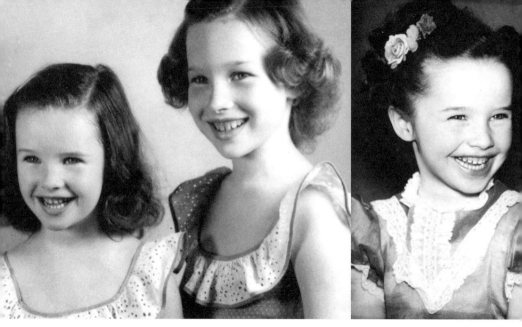

My sister, Judy, right, always looked out for me. She was concerned that no one made life rough for her little sister. Mother made our dresses.

Mother always dressed me nicely and put ribbons or flowers in my hair.

I had an active grade school life. I did not enjoy most summer camps I attended until I became a Girl Scout and went with the other girls in the troop to an incredible camp. The counselor at the camp was a student at Oklahoma City University (OCU), my first introduction to the university that would become so much a part of my life.

Music and church were integral parts of my young life. Mother always expected Judy and me to sing in the children's choir. It was very clear to us that she considered all gifts from God should be used for His purpose and His glory. It was not negotiable whether or not we sang first in the children's choir and then in the adult choir at First Methodist Church. Karen Self and Carolyn Fry were older than me, but became great friends through our participation in church activities, especially in our weekly Methodist Youth Fellowship (MYF) meetings.

My sister, Judy, had perfect pitch and could arrange music at an early age. While she was still in grade school, she formed a girls quartet that sang all over southwestern Oklahoma. Music was even part of our basketball trips. I will never forget the students singing the hymn, "Living for Jesus,"

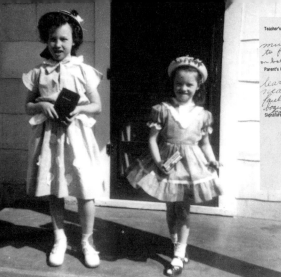

Because my mother was my fifth grade teacher, she had to complete both the "teacher's comment" and "parent's comment" on the back of my report card. I made all A's except for writing, prompting mother to write, "Janie can write much neater and needs to form the habit now." In the parent's comment, mother wrote, "It is the teacher's fault—I'm going to see the board about a new fifth grade teacher. You should make the children happy with all A's." Mother has always had such a great sense of humor.

Judy, left, and me ready for Sunday School. Mother made certain we never missed Sunday services and we always carried our Bibles to church.

in four-part harmony, before each game. I can remember sitting beside my mother on our way to games, feeling the coldness of the school bus, the warmth of my mother, and the sound of that precious hymn being sung so beautifully by the players and cheerleaders.

Judy and I used music for every occasion. One dark night after a movie, she was walking me home. As we headed up a hill, the darkness and shadows of usually familiar neighborhoods became distorted by our feelings of fear. We sensed the change and Judy reached for my scardy-cat hand. "Let's sing," she said. She always took charge and made me feel safe.

So two little voices tuned up in the night with hesitation and self-consciousness at first, but with increasing volume and heart. "When you walk through a storm, keep your head up high, and don't be afraid of the dark. At the end of the storm, there's a golden sky and the sweet silver song of the lark." With each phrase our voices grew stronger, we held our heads higher, and our steps were more courageous.

My early spiritual growth, in addition to excellent training at home, came from the longtime pastor at First Methodist Church, Reverend

Leonard Gillingham and his wife, Martha. Reverend Gillingham had a gift of encouragement. When I was at church camp at Devil's Canyon, I would always receive a note from the pastor, with words of encouragement such as, "I sure hope you have a deep experience with God this week. I know you will."

Reverend Gillingham was an extraordinary human being who played a major role in my life long after his assignment in Sentinel was completed. Another pastor, Reverend Sanford Wylie, was also special primarily because he brought me a new best friend, his daughter, Barbara. We often sang in church. One of the most embarrassing moments in my early teen years was when Barbara and I were singing a duet, "Star of the East," and could not stop laughing. Here was a teacher's kid and the preacher's kid laughing hysterically while trying to sing a serious religious song. No matter how many glares my mother gave us, or how upset her father was, we could not control our laughing.

I did not realize it at the time, but my faith in God was being nourished by teaching at church and at home, and also by every day occurrences in life. One of my first memories of the concept of grace was during an old-fashioned ice cream church social. There was holiness surrounding such an occasion that was unrecognizable to me as a child, but so obvious now.

On a summer night, with the scene of freshly mowed grass, the coolness of a light breeze, and the mixture of insect sounds and laughter, the families gathered in the grassy area next to the church. Parishioners arrived on the lawn burdened with ice cream freezers packed with salt and ice. Inside the freezer was the luscious cream that would soon be frozen by cranking the handle.

Small children like me sat on the top of piles of towels or rugs covering the freezer. The extra weight seemed to make the process of salt melting the ice work its magic quickly. We knew the ice cream was "done" when the crank would hardly turn. The anticipation of the tastes of that summer sweetness was almost more than we could stand.

After the ice cream was frozen, it was spooned out into bowls. Before the children could be captured by adults, we scattered into a nearby yard to sit on a big quilt and eat our heavenly treat. As night fell, we observed the starry sky, the vastness and beauty of God's creation. It seemed that God was within reach, the same as the love of a church community and the personal security of my family. We were all so small compared to the incredible creation of sky and space. But inside my young heart, I knew I was somehow connected to it all. It was too spectacular to be happenstance. It was too personally significant to be superficial. The presence of God and his awesome grace was all there. We did not know what to call that feeling, but it was grace nonetheless.

Judy and I not only liked to sing, we greatly enjoyed dancing. We could hardly wait to watch "American Bandstand" and dance in front of the television set. We learned to dance with each other and all our cousins who learned the same way.

My mother has often said that I was not a simple child to raise. I was not difficult, but she knew from the beginning that I was more complex than some children. I was such a dreamer and loved the idea of performing. My dolls, dressed in exquisite gowns, were always in mythical pageants. At the same time, I was very much a tomboy. I hated shopping and frilly clothing. I got a huge kick out of telling my dad when my mother and Judy went shopping.

I hated curly hair. Mother gave us home permanents until we began driving to Mountain View for a hairdresser to put lots of curls in our hair. I could hold my own with my male friends at school or church, whether it was in a discussion about the Bible or just playing.

My mother's influence in my life extended far beyond the classroom and at home. She was a church choir leader, taught Bible school and Sunday school, and helped with my Brownies group before I became a full-fledged Girl Scout.

Daddy was always interested in giving his family the best he could afford. We attended many University of Oklahoma (OU) football games and attended high school sporting events almost weekly. Daddy was also our early storm warning system. He was decades ahead of radio and television weathermen in predicting a coming storm. He watched the clouds closely while we played cards or read books. It was a time of excitement, especially when he would yell, "It's time to hit the cellar!" We then bundled up, grabbed he dog, and descended into the cellar in the back yard until the storm passed.

My junior high years were not great. I struggled because there were so few girls in my class, and most of them lived outside town. I loved playing girls' basketball and singing at every opportunity, in school or church.

Our social life had always been enriched by the great friendships among my parents' friends. We spent many meals together and had hours of fun. Family friends in Sentinel included School Superintendent Clarence Overstreet and his wife, Quay, Dr. Aubrey and Mary Stowers, J.C. and Geneva Farris, Hayden and Ruby Lee Webb, and Mary and Charles McClure.

We moved into a new house in Sentinel after daddy and his brother built a few houses to sell. Our house was the one that did not sell. Judy and I were thrilled because the new house had a half-bath, a fifty percent increase in bathroom space for four people, including two teenage girls.

I started liking boys in junior high school, although I made some poor choices. I was in trouble much of the time. My parents would not allow me to date until I was 16 so my friends would try to get around that rule by meeting boys at the movie and getting in their cars afterwards. Once, daddy found us. I was humiliated and in a lot of trouble. I also once dated a boy who was in town for harvest. He kept me out way past my curfew, and I was grounded again. I am grateful daddy was a tough disciplinarian.

When I was not dreaming of boys, I had my nose in a book. I was an avid reader and a frequent visitor to both the school and town libraries. I still have a certificate for reading 60 books in the sixth grade. My vivid imagination was exploited in reading books such as *My Friend Flicka, Black Beauty, Heidi,* and *Little Women.*

My affection for music grew one fall when we attended my first musical, *Calamity Jane,* starring Carol Burnett, in Dallas, Texas, where we had traveled for the annual football battle between OU and the University of Texas. I was so taken with the musical. As the curtain closed and the applause rose, daddy suggested we try to beat the crowd and leave. But I could not. I was crying, so thrilled at how musical theater had impacted my soul. Deep in my heart, I dreamed that I could someday perform on a stage like that. As usual, my parents saw how I was affected, so we were the last people to leave the theater. I had been touched by the magic and musical theater remains one of my greatest joys.

My sister and I took piano lessons for what seemed like forever. One of our teachers was Mabel Cauthron who insisted we practice several hours each day. Fern Howard and later, Mel Keeney, were important music teachers as well. Mother agreed that Judy and I needed to practice—she even offered to take our place doing the dishes after supper. If we took a night off, and did the dishes ourselves, we still used music to pass the time by. Often, as Judy handed me a wet plate to dry, we would harmonize on "Singing in the Rain," so loudly that our parents were aware of our antics in the other room.

Judy graduated as valedictorian of her class at Sentinel High School in 1960. She was everything—she played basketball and was a great musician and performer. She was offered a full scholarship to OCU, largely because she held a statewide office in the Methodist Youth Fellowship. However, when she went to Dallas for a visit with Aunt Honore and Uncle John

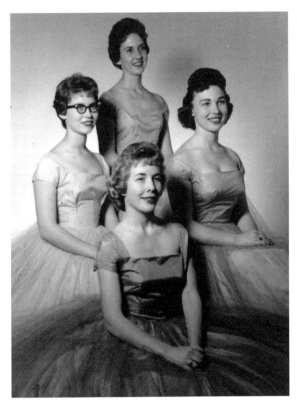

My sister, Judy, and three of her friends sang all over western Oklahoma. Left to right, Judy Sanderlin, Sandra Self, and Judy. In front is Pat Walker, who named her daughter, Jayne, after me in 1959.

Mitchell, she fell in love with Southern Methodist University (SMU). My parents agreed she could attend college at SMU if she could get a scholarship and a part-time job. She did.

With Judy's graduation from high school, it was a time of transition for our family. Daddy had coached Judy in high school basketball but wanted to use his master's degree in school administration. He took a job as junior high principal in Laverne, Oklahoma. Also, dad had great respect for Harry Shackleford, the Laverne superintendent of schools.

Needless to say, it was a traumatic time for me, leaving the only place I had ever lived and moving to Laverne the summer before my freshman year in high school. Daddy and mother made every effort to make our move to Laverne smooth. I went from a class size of 17 to 65 students. One of the pluses about moving to a larger school district, my parents said, was that I could be in a marching band. So before we left Sentinel, I was allowed to buy a saxophone. Mother also drove me for months to Hobart to take lessons to learn to play the instrument.

I arrived in Laverne with a good feeling, that the move was absolutely divine providence. I learned from my parents that Laverne, in western Harper County, was named for Laverne Smith, a local resident of the village when the post office was established on March 30, 1898.

The good thing about being in a larger school system was that I went from having so many things come easily to having to work for everything I achieved. However, that blessing was not readily apparent to me on the day in August of my 14th year when I appeared for my first meeting with the Laverne High School marching band. I suddenly realized I did not know how to march!

Going into a new group of kids was already worse than having the flu. But on that first day of band practice, the director ushered band members onto Main Street to practice marching. The drum major raised her arms, blew her whistle three times, and off we went, or I should say, off they went. I stumbled and tried to follow students around me. Then there was another whistle, a command of which I knew nothing, and I stumbled some more. I bumped into my neighbors and was mortified. I knew the eyes of every member of the band were focused on me.

There was only one thing to do—run! With saxophone in hand, I ran home, crying every inch of the way. I never wanted to go back. I was totally embarrassed. As usual, my family was wonderful. Daddy said, "Well, I can teach you how to march. I learned in the Navy." Mom had marched in a high school band also knew how to march. Judy was up for anything. To diffuse the devastation of the moment, we marched around inside the house until my sadness turned to laughter. My heart was so full, not from pain, from the joy of knowing I had my family.

No matter what else—a new school, a new house, a new town—I had my family. All things could change, but not the love they had for me. What an anchor!

My mother was such a positive influence. The first time I ever remember her being in the audience was when I played a non-speaking role as Christopher Robin in a school play. My role was a sleeping child who just lay in the middle of a group of children. But as I lay there with all the tension and apprehension of a first stage appearance, I opened my eyes just enough to gaze at the audience and feel the bright lights and experience the attention that is directed at performers. I liked it!

Another change for me when we moved to Laverne was the "y" change in my first name. After seeing my first musical in Dallas and watching the Miss America Pageant annually, I had dreams of seeing my name in print or on a marquee. I had always liked my double initials, although I preferred the more sophisticated sounding "Jane" over "Janie," but I had little control over what adults called me. At least "Janie" was better than calling me "Pedro" because I sometimes wore dog ears.

How cool would it be to add a "y" to the "Jane" and make my name even more attractive in print? So when we moved to Laverne, I became "Jayne' Jayroe, and even though I continued to be "Janie," I always wrote "Jayne" which explains the confusion over the spelling of my name in later years.

When I began applying for colleges, I was feeling much more humble at the thought of leaving my small town cocoon of support, and I also needed a name to match my birth certificate. I did not want anything in the application process to bring attention to me. So, I changed my name back to plain "Jane," but the "y" continues to stick today. I love it both ways.

Mother always found some way to praise each of my performances, whether on the basketball court or on stage. After a piano recital at an early age, she said, "You seem to feel the music so much." "You were the prettiest one," she might say with a smile after I played a lousy basketball game." That was a joke between us because she knew I was surely the only girl on the starting lineup who slept in curlers and spent a lot of time on my hair and makeup before a game. Our star players were outstanding young women who lived on farms and wore little or no makeup. "Being the prettiest one" was not a competition they were interested in, so the comment was a little fun between mother and me.

Mother always urged me to try my best, but she never pushed me. She could help me absorb any disappointment, and was never embarrassed by my efforts. It was expected that I would do the right thing and be responsible and nice. The high standards of performance were my own making.

Laverne was such a great place for me in the early 1960s because I was in a class of overachievers and had to work for everything. Yet there was an opportunity to participate in every activity—music contests, Future Homemakers of America, cheerleading, band, choir, rainbow for girls, church choir, journalism projects, basketball, and Methodist Youth Fellowship.

It seemed as if I was always competing in something. It was great for character building to learn to lose and try again, to experience a "1" or win, and to share a common dream with a team of other people. There were great lessons learned about life in Laverne. We were wrapped in a community of supportive families who knew your name, attended your basketball games, saw you at church, and applauded you at graduation. I am so glad I was Miss America FROM Laverne, Oklahoma. It was an honor shared by the good folks of a great town.

REVEREND LEONARD GILLINGHAM

~ ~ ~ *"Janie was a bright young girl who loved to sing in church and help her mother in church projects. She had a contagious smile and worked very hard to excel in every way."*

DAVID WALTERS

~ ~ ~ *"As a high school junior I admired from afar this young beauty who had just become Miss America. Since I was growing up in Canute, it was not lost on me that she was from another small Oklahoma town. 'Anything is possible,' I thought. Later as governor, when I got to know Jane, it was special. That smile, those piercing eyes, great wit, and sharp mind definitely kept me focused. Every recent governor appointed Jane to something. In my case, it was to the very unglamorous position on the Legislative Compensation Board. I was convinced that her infectious smile would calm those who inevitably get upset no matter what the board does. Raise salaries and make voters mad—don't raise salaries and legislators get mad. Jane handled the assignment with her usual grace."*

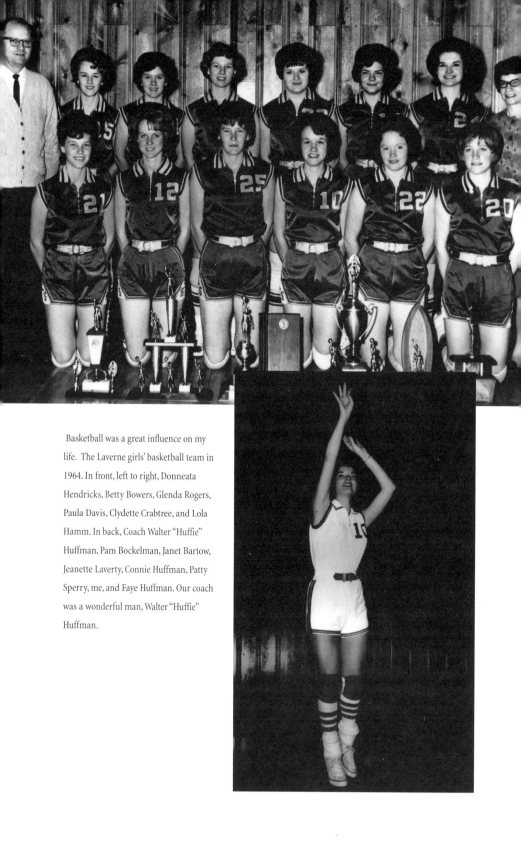

Basketball was a great influence on my life. The Laverne girls' basketball team in 1964. In front, left to right, Donneata Hendricks, Betty Bowers, Glenda Rogers, Paula Davis, Clydette Crabtree, and Lola Hamm. In back, Coach Walter "Huffie" Huffman, Pam Bockelman, Janet Bartow, Jeanette Laverty, Connie Huffman, Patty Sperry, me, and Faye Huffman. Our coach was a wonderful man, Walter "Huffie" Huffman.

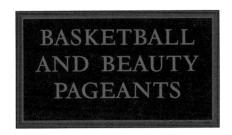

4

BASKETBALL AND BEAUTY PAGEANTS

ven though my family made the move to Laverne easier, I was a basket case on the first day of school. I had gone to the same school in Sentinel my entire life, now I was being driven to a new school with new people. When my mother, who was also going to a new teaching assignment in a new school, drove me to Laverne High School, I refused to get out of the car.

I did not want to go in the building. The superintendent's son, Jimmy Shackleford, and the girl's basketball coach, Walt Huffman's daughter, Connie, had both been nice to me. But it did not matter—I did not want to go in. Mother was getting upset at me because she did not want to be late for her first day of class. She finally pushed me out of the car and I headed for the building.

To make matters worse, the first person I saw was Lynn Hoch, a nice looking young man for whom I had developed a huge crush during my first few weeks in Laverne. When I saw Lynn with his girlfriend, Janie Wyand, I dropped everything in my hands. After that embarrassing moment, the rest of the day was anti-climactic.

What a wonderful group of freshmen classmates I had. Lynn, Lulu Wofford, Janet Bartow, Bob Hickman, and Jimmy Shackleford all later went to college and became outstanding leaders in their respective professions and great citizens.

I was so busy on football game days because I was a cheerleader and played in the band. Before a home game, I cheered at the pep assembly, decorated the goal posts at the football stadium, and ran home to change into-my cheerleader uniform for the game. Just before halftime, I ran into the cold restroom and changed into my band uniform for the halftime show. Then, I changed back into my cheerleader uniform for the remainder of the game. I knew nothing about football except whether we were winning or losing.

Football was a popular sport in Laverne but there was no question that girls' basketball was king, or queen, of the culture in the town. The Laverne girls' program was one of the premier programs in Oklahoma.

The girls on my team had been together since the fifth grade and were determined to win the state tournament. They had trained together and knew each other's move on the court, both in practice and during games. Two of the girls I played with, Lola Hamm and Glenda Rogers, were named All-State players and went on to play after graduation. Glenda played on the Pan American team and Lola received a full scholarship to Wayland Baptist University in Plainview, Texas. I worked hard to make the first team—and eventually did. I loved playing for Coach Walter "Huffie" Huffman who was also a great friend of my parents and a wonderful human being.

In addition to enjoying the benefits of an outstanding basketball legacy at Laverne, I also sat under the teaching of excellent instructors. Keith Ann Armor, my English teacher, was my first instructor who required me to think in a creative way. I had always assumed that writing a good paper was just following correct grammatical rules. Mrs. Armor pushed me to think and write creatively. For the first time, I had to work hard to make good grades.

Another outstanding teacher was Alma Bartow, my instructor in biology and chemistry. She was a very serious teacher, not impressed with cheerleaders or musical performers. She had nothing against that type of girl, she just thought science was the most important thing in the world. When Mrs. Bartow awarded me a special science award, I think we both were surprised. Unfortunately, there was no vocal music program at Laverne. Mother tried to support my interests with private lessons.

At 15, I was super interested in boys. Daddy had a strict rule that his girls could not date until age 16, a rule that was out of line with Laverne culture because younger teenagers often walked together to the movie or Teen

Town. My mother and sister went to bat for me and daddy finally gave in. I was allowed to date six months before my 16th birthday.

Three major things happened to me during my sophomore year in high school. I was named homecoming queen, I was maid of honor in my sister's wedding to Don Wieser, a young football coach at Laverne High School—and I met Jimmy Webb.

Jimmy was the son of a Baptist preacher who moved his family to Laverne to become pastor of the local Baptist congregation. Reverend Webb preached against dancing, so those of us who attended Teen Town on Friday nights to dance did not have a good first impression of him.

Jimmy was not cool. He was tall and skinny and wore large black-rimmed glasses that were always sliding down on his nose. But he could play the piano! The oldest of four children, Jimmy had been taught to play piano by his mother. Jimmy was an absent minded musical genius. His father, a great athlete in his time, made him try out for football and basketball.

Daddy, knowing that Jimmy was anything but a gifted basketball player, took the youngster under his wing. They really liked each other. Daddy even taught Jimmy in drivers education, a big challenge.

Jimmy and I shared a love for music so he spent many afternoons and evenings at our home. Often, his mother would call our house to tell mother to send Jimmy home.

Like me, Jimmy was a dreamer. He would tell me about a musical or score for a movie he was writing in his head. Then, to prove he was not just talk, he would play the music for me. In my scrapbooks are many songs written by Jimmy, songs that never made it to the top of American music charts when he later wrote huge hits such as "Up, Up, and Away," "By the Time I Get to Phoenix," "Wichita Lineman," and "MacArthur Park."

At our sophomore assembly, I sang "I Understand," a Jimmy Webb composition that contained all the elements of his later successful commercial hits. The first two verses of the song were classic Jimmy:

I understand just how you feel,
Your love for me might not be real,
It's over now but it was grand,
I understand, I understand.

If you ever change your mind,
Come back to me,
And you will find,
Me waiting there, at your command.
I understand, I understand.

Another of Jimmy's high school compositions that we sang together was "Just Excuse the Slip." The music and lyrics were far beyond his tender years:

If when I hold your hand my love,
I hold it much too tight,
You'll have to understand, my love,
If I don't kiss you right.

For I haven't held many hands, dear love,
I haven't kissed many lips,
And should I hold you too tight my love,
Just Excuse the Slip.

Jimmy was like a brother to me. We sang so much together, we became quite a performing team for everyone in the Laverne area. As long as Jimmy would play, I would sing for almost any occasion. We sang at school assemblies, weddings, and just about anywhere people were gathered and needed entertainment.

In our junior year, Joy Seiger Mahan's sister, Alma Jo Weinmeister, heard us perform and was determined that Jimmy and I have careers in performing arts. She drove us to Oklahoma City in her Cadillac to audition for Tom Paxton, the host of a very popular variety show on an Oklahoma City television station. Unfortunately, Paxton and his people did not think we had sufficient talent to be on the local television show. Ironically, Jimmy was only a few years from penning, at age 19, his first national number one song, "Up, Up, and Away," recorded by the Fifth Dimension, and I was only a few years away from being crowned Miss America.

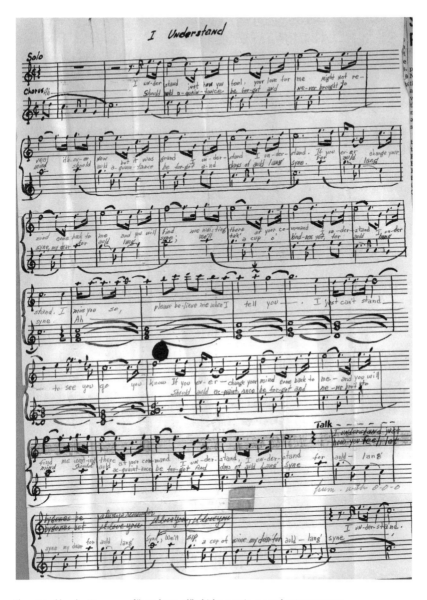

The original handwritten score of "I Understand," which I sang in our sophomore program.

After the turn-down at the television station, Alma Jo drove us to a downtown Oklahoma City recording studio where we recorded a two-song record, both Jimmy's compositions. On one side was "Grey Skies are Better than Blue When I'm Underneath Them With You." On the other side of the record was "Please Excuse The Slip."

Jimmy's family moved to California after his junior year at Laverne. His mother died soon after that, a tragedy for all of them. She was the one who understood her genius son the most and left the world a gift in his ability. When Jimmy's father moved back to Oklahoma, Jimmy stayed in California and became a superstar in the music industry.

I am so proud of my lifelong friendship with Jimmy. In his 35 years of success, he is the only artist to ever receive Grammy awards for music, lyrics, and orchestration. "By The Time I Get to Phoenix" is the third most performed song in the last 50 years. His songs have been made into hits by Glen Campbell, Richard Harris, the Fifth Dimension, the Brooklyn Bridge, Linda Ronstadt, Joe Crocker, Waylon Jennings, Willie Nelson, Johnny Cash, and Kris Kristofferson.

Jimmy, after having five top ten hits within a 20-month period in the 1960s, was called "new genius" by the music world. Frank Sinatra declared "By The Time I Get to Phoenix" the "greatest torch song ever written" and said he enjoyed singing Jimmy's songs because "he has been blessed with the emotions and artistic talent of the great lyricists."

Jimmy has influenced a new generation of songwriters. Billy Joel credits Jimmy as a major influence in his career. In his book about songwriting, Jimmy says, "The paramount joy of the craft is that, however simply it is begun, it can take the songwriter on a lifelong voyage across many distant and wondrous musical seas."

Jimmy and I had a very special relationship. Growing up for him was difficult, which probably only added to his artistic depth. He was a musical genius and yet he was not easily accepted into the small rural school culture. I would like to believe I was understanding, but I was pretty busy being popular myself.

I liked Jimmy and loved sharing his music. While I knew his talent was beyond anything I had experienced, I could not imagine that he would have such success so early in life.

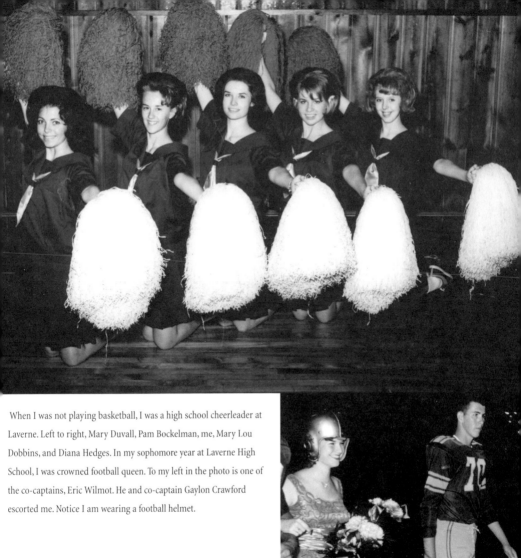

When I was not playing basketball, I was a high school cheerleader at Laverne. Left to right, Mary Duvall, Pam Bockelman, me, Mary Lou Dobbins, and Diana Hedges. In my sophomore year at Laverne High School, I was crowned football queen. To my left in the photo is one of the co-captains, Eric Wilmot. He and co-captain Gaylon Crawford escorted me. Notice I am wearing a football helmet.

God works in mysterious ways. Had the Webb family not moved to California, who knows if Jimmy would have had the kind of early success—putting him in the right place at the right time.

There were moments in high school, when Jimmy was playing our little piano in a renovated garage, that I had a glimpse into his future greatness. It was quite an emotional high to be able to sit on a piano bench with him and enter into the edge of his superior world of music. It was a privilege to be part of something so creative.

When I was not practicing or performing with Jimmy, I was in the high school gymnasium playing basketball. I can remember the feeling of flying around the basketball court like it was yesterday. There is nothing like the exhilaration of being in shape, being part of a dedicated team of athletes, and wanting the goal of a championship.

In my four years of high school competition, we lost only four or five games total. We were awesome. We loved the game. We respected the coach. We thrilled over winning. And we trained like there was no other way.

We practiced every day with the coach during the season, and worked out on our own during the off season. We kept strict curfew hours. We never smoked nor drank alcohol. We hardly dated—preparing and discipline was everything. We meant business.

In my junior year, our girls' basketball team was good enough to win the state championship. However, on a disputed call, we lost in the regional tournament to Fairview at their home court. There was a huge disagreement as to whether Fairview's winning basket was made before the final buzzer. The poor timekeeper, an employee of the Fairview school system, had to make the call, and it went to the advantage of Fairview.

In my senior year, we made it all the way to the state championship game against Mangum. In the second overtime, with only seconds remaining, I fouled Greta Hogan, whose successful free throw was the difference in the game. My teammates never blamed me, a fact confirmed in a Newsweek magazine article written about me after I was Miss America. The coach was quoted in Newsweek, "Janie was part of the team, and the other five Tigerettes were as much a part of the loss as Janie."

My first entry into a beauty pageant came during my senior year in the Miss Cinderella pageant at Northwestern State College in Alva. I had passionately watched the Miss America pageant for as long as I could remember and openly cried with joy when the winner was named each year. My dad always kidded me because I cried more than the girl who won. I was deeply moved by the Miss America pageant, and somehow knew I wanted to compete someday.

The Miss Cinderella pageant at Northwestern was used to publicize the school as part of its annual homecoming celebration. They asked surrounding towns to send representatives to the contest. The Laverne Chamber of Commerce decided one of the town's beauties should enter the pageant so it sponsored a pageant. I was one of 12 girls who entered the Miss Laverne pageant.

It was a decision that would either affirm my dream of majoring in music in college and seeking a career in music, or force me to major in chemistry, which I really liked, and take a totally different career route.

For my talent in the Miss Laverne pageant, I chose the song, "With a Song in My Heart," from the Jane Froman story that became a hit movie. I always liked the movie because it was set in World War II and my father and all my uncles had served in the military. Froman, after being injured, continued to perform for soldiers. She was such a hero to me.

I knew that if I could sing well enough to win a contest, maybe I could attend Oklahoma City University and sing in the Surrey Singers. I certainly was not brave like my sister and would never have gone out of state to college. I was a momma's girl and wanted to stay close to home.

I practiced hard and won the Miss Laverne contest and prepared for the competition at Northwestern. My accompanist was my sister, Judy, who was very pregnant at the time. My mother and Judy made my dress with the help of Luisa Evans, a wonderful Austrian seamstress in Laverne.

We went to Alva early to visit our dear friends and number one supporters Madeline Argenbright and her daughter Annie. Who knew that Annie would be Miss Cinderella in later years?

Mother was my chaperone at a dinner with the judges before the competition. I tried to do everything perfectly. I kept putting my knife at the top of my plate like I thought I was supposed to do, but it kept falling off. The sound reverberated throughout the room. I thought surely everyone noticed me, an uncouth and unsophisticated high school girl from Laverne.

The judges must have not heard my knife-clanking, because I was named Miss Cinderella 1963, chosen from a field of 23 girls in the contest. I was so excited.

As usual, my mother was in the audience when I won my first beauty crown. Mother was always there for me. In fact, I took it for granted she would be there. It was as if there was a special spiritual presence that came

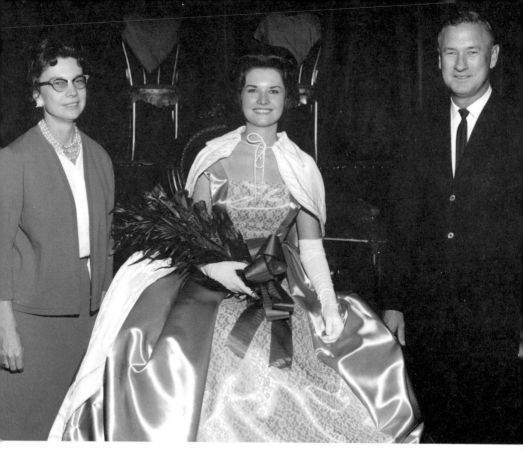

Mother and Daddy pose with me after the Miss Cinderella pageant in Alva.

from her spot in the audience to my spot on the stage. It was an energy I depended upon. When my deepest fears set in, I knew she was there. When I was afraid I would look foolish, I knew she was there. When I would forget the words, I knew she was there. When I would miss the goal, I knew she was there. And when I would feel like a star, I knew she was there.

After I won the Miss Cinderella contest, I talked my sister's ear off for hours. She was only a few weeks from giving birth to her first child and was obviously tired and needed sleep. After the show, I promised to give her any of my prizes she wanted, if she would just stay awake and listen to me chatter. She was exhausted and kept falling sleep as I was bouncing around.

My classmates could not be at my coronation as Miss Cinderella, because Laverne played Beaver in football that night. However, I knew all my friends would flock around me the next day at a band contest in Alva. When I arrived, expecting everyone to suffocate me with their attention, I was totally snubbed. Some of my friends circulated rumors that I won because my mother knew the judges. That was absurd!

Ironically, because of winning the beauty pageant, I lost most of my good friends during my senior year in high school. However, their loss was my gain—I drew closer to three extraordinary people, Lennie "LuLu" Wofford, her sister, Janie, and Bob Hickman. LuLu was an outstanding student and drum major of our band. She loved politics and baseball and was so supportive of me. Bob was my boyfriend and had been one of my best friends all the years at Laverne. My parents loved him, a plus for any high school romantic relationship. Eventually, our lives took different directions and he married a fellow cheerleader and an outstanding woman, Mary Lou Dobbins.

I never held any grudges against my former friends who dropped me after I won the beauty pageant. For high school girls, shunning other girls is unfortunately not an uncommon phenomenon, but it is hurtful.

I was so blessed with my immediate family that provided great insulation to the rocky road of my last year in high school. My extended family also was important. We attended most OU-Texas weekends and summer vacations with grandparents and cousins. The Christmas holiday was special. Mama May renovated her garage at her home in Enid into a room that could accommodate many grandchildren.

The "big people" ate in the dining room and the kids ate in the kitchen. We never had any problems—we just enjoyed having a dozen or so cousins around, playing games and loving every minute of it. A special treat was the fun that our parents had during the family reunions, staying up all hours of the night playing cards. It was a great legacy to drift off to sleep at night with the laughter of our parents ringing in our ears.

Our family grew in November, 1963, when my sister gave birth to her first son, Jace Don Wieser. It was a great event. I was a senior in high school and a devoted aunt—I still am. Jace became part of our entourage. Wherever I was performing, Judy and I dragged the baby along.

BILL ARMOUR

~ ~ ~ *"During Janie's high school years, I taught the high school Sunday School class at the Laverne Methodist Church. She was a faithful member and never missed unless there was a good reason. I especially remember one winter day when a heavy snow made travel difficult. I walked to church to be there in case any other brave soul ventured out of their homes. Only one person showed up that day—Jane Ann. She took her religion quite seriously, even as a young person. Jane's personality and goodness has propelled her far beyond Laverne. But when she comes home, she is friendly to all, old timers and newcomers. I remember one humorous incident. Jane took in a good deal of money during her year as Miss America. I prepared her tax return, and sure enough, she received notice of an audit by the Internal Revenue Service. Because of her heavy schedule, Jane could not go to meet the auditor at the Woodward, Oklahoma IRS office. Her father, Pete, and I made the appointment where we met a young auditor who was very disappointed that Miss America was not there for the audit."*

ANNA MILLERET

~ ~ ~ *"Jane and I have a deep spiritual bond that comes from the seed of our mother's faith and our parents' friendship. She is my kindred spirit. I shall never forget being fascinated by this feminine brunette beauty fiercely playing basketball with her hair coifed in a French roll. You could see the bobby pins flying as she galloped across the field house."*

LENNIE "LULU" WOFFORD STEINBRINK

~ ~ ~ Janie and I became fast friends when she moved to
Laverne. She became part of every activity and club in town.
Laverne was a wonderful place to grow up in the 1960s and we
enjoyed an idyllic teenage life. Jane is a loyal and loving person,
much like her mother and sister. They are always positive
and are 'givers.' "

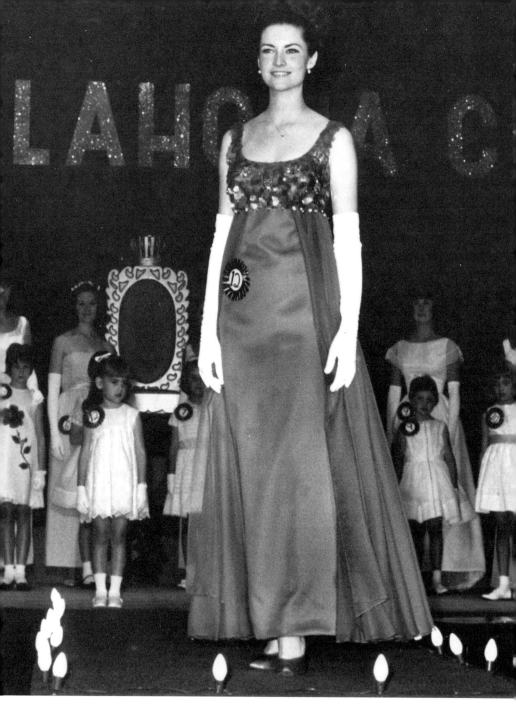

I was a little nervous in the evening gown competition in the Miss Oklahoma City Pageant, especially in my green dress.

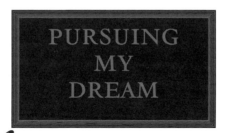

PURSUING MY DREAM

When I graduated from high school in 1964, I had options of where I would attend college. One of the prizes of winning the Miss Cinderella contest at Northwestern State College at Alva was a four-year scholarship to the school. My parents were, of course, thrilled with the prospect of the scholarship. But I could not give up on my dream to attend OCU in Oklahoma City. I believed it was God's calling for me to pursue a music degree at OCU.

The university was located on 55 acres at the corner of Northwest 23rd Street and Blackwelder Avenue in Oklahoma City. The school began in 1904 as Epworth University, the dream of a young Edmond, Oklahoma, attorney, Anton H. Classen. He was a dedicated Methodist and worked diligently to promote a Methodist school of higher learning for Oklahoma City. Known as Methodist University and Oklahoma City College for several years, the school was given its present name in 1923.

My parents were completely supportive but could not financially afford to pay full tuition and room and board at the private Methodist school. My only alternative was to apply for scholarships to supplement my parents' assistance. Fortunately, I was awarded a partial scholarship and a work study opportunity in the journalism department. I was frugal with my $10 a month allowance from my parents. I thanked them profusely for giving me the chance to pursue my dream.

I was a little afraid to leave home, although Oklahoma City really was not that far from Laverne. When I arrived on campus at OCU, I knew no one. I was lucky to be assigned a perfect roommate, Deanna Owens from Stroud, Oklahoma. We were very different in many ways, but a perfect combination as good friends and roommates.

I had no problem making new friends, but I was terribly homesick and missed my mother. I struggled the entire first semester, but made a relatively quick adjustment, largely because the professors at OCU were so caring and the students so friendly.

I was both surprised and elated at the difficulty of my studies in the music school at OCU. My piano teacher, Nancy Apgar, and my legendary voice teacher, Inez Silberg, were very demanding. I knew I did not have the vocal skills of many of my fellow students, but Mrs. Silberg took me as serious as if I had an opera career around the corner. She requested I be an accompanist for other voice students so I would be exposed to more than one lesson each week. Mrs. Apgar treated me like a piano major, although I was taking the class as a requirement for a degree in vocal music education.

I made wonderful friends at OCU—Cinde Eide of Oklahoma City, Susan Thompson of Calumet, Oklahoma, and Janice Steele of Tulsa. They wanted me to join their sorority, Alpha Chi Omega. I frankly knew very little about sororities and had not participated in rush. My friends gathered information about me and somehow arranged for me to be in their pledge class. Sharon Albert was our pledge trainer and helped me make the transition. Tracy Thompson was our president and my idol. She was beautiful, kind, and full of grace.

Sororities are different at OCU. Girls live in the dormitory and eat in the student cafeteria, rather than living in a sorority house off campus. Our sorority meetings were held in an apartment on campus. The group of friends I made in my sorority made the transition to college much easier. Another good friend, Tresa Hall, was president of a different sorority, Gamma Phi Beta. We called her "Texas," because she grew up in Atlanta, Texas. My best friend in the music school, Sue Wells, was also a Gamma Phi.

My sorority sisters knew of my involvement in the Miss Cinderella pageant in high school, so they sponsored me as a participant in the contest for All College Queen for the All College Basketball Tournament held each Christmas season in Oklahoma City. I found a bright green $50 evening gown at Shepherd Mall in Oklahoma City and asked my parents if the dress could be my early Christmas present. They agreed, because competing in a beauty pageant at a basketball tournament was the best of both worlds for a true basketball family. The judges included Ross Porter, Ken Kerrigan, and Lois Evans, chair of the Miss Oklahoma City pageant. To my surprise, I won. It was a wonderful experience to be crowned All College Basketball Queen on center court of the Oklahoma City Civic Center. Two of the other finalists, Linda Duncan Talkington and Bobbi Ingram Moore, remain friends today.

As a freshman music student, the performance opportunities were limited at OCU. The music department was very opera oriented, but the production of *The Crucible,* at least gave me the chance to perform. Janie Zerger, one of my idols, was one of the leads in the opera. Judy Schultz and Bob Pappas also had leading roles. Sue Wells and I were double cast for the smallest role in the production. Even though it was at best a bit part, it was a great experience to be around people for which I such great respect.

For rehearsals, Sue and I had to stay at school during spring break. Because the school cafeteria was closed, we drove to Quick's for a quarter hamburger every night and ate soup and popcorn for that week. We had little money to dine anywhere else. She performed the role one night, and I performed the next. The thrill was being on the same stage with Janie Zerger.

All vocal music students were required to sing in the OCU choir under the direction of Professor Archie Brown. Hearing my voice raised with all the other voices was thrilling to me. It suited me perfectly to sing in a choir. My friends knew I was shy, so they expected me to want to sing only in a large group. They often accused me of being so shy that I just stood around at social functions and smiled. That was the way I handled stress or self-consciousness—a trait that helped me later on in pageants.

I was not one of the best voices in the school of music, but I did work very hard and practiced as much as the professors recommended. I was fortunate to have several opportunities to perform. Keshena Kapers, a Greek system competition of musical skits, gave me the chance to perform and work with my friends in the sorority and school of music. I had great regard for Emogene Collins, my Italian diction teacher, and the incredible Florence Birdwell who had just begun to teach voice at OCU.

At the end of the school year, I wanted to audition for Lyric Theater in Oklahoma City, but also wanted to go home. I put off the Lyric dream and spent the summer in Laverne.

Even though mine was not an opera voice, and my performing opportunities were few and far between, my experience at the OCU music school was terrific. I was treated with as much seriousness as Leona Mitchell who was a few years behind me. Leona, who has become a world-renowned opera star, was a sweet girl and was very close to my best friend, Sue Wells.

My only disappointment during my sophomore year at OCU was failing to land a spot in the Surrey Singers, a singing group that traveled around the country and even sang in USO tours, one of my goals in life, going all the way back to the Jane Fromann movie. I was devastated when the participants of Surrey Singers did not select me at their audition. OCU's School of Music had an international reputation and the people I competed against had great voices. I did realize that maybe my voice was not on that level, but surely my stage presence made up for it. Apparently, it did not. Sue Wells did make it, and another of my best friends in the music school, Don Johnson, was the accompanist for the Surrey Singers. Don was off the chart in terms of his musical ability.

After losing the opportunity to be part of the Surrey Singers, I questioned God, "What have you called me to do?" I thought singing and performing was my calling. God replaced the desire to sing with the Surrey Singers quickly. Looking back, the admonition, "Oh ye of little faith," certainly applied to me. I had no ideas what plans God had in store for me.

Within that month, Dolly Hoskins, one of the preliminary judges in the All College Queen competition, suggested I enter the Miss Oklahoma City pageant. Dolly was director of the pageant. Suggest is probably the wrong word, because Dolly called me several times and pressured me into entering the pageant. My sorority friends were so encouraging, a far cry from the reaction of my friends when I won a high school beauty pageant. I agreed to enter, but strictly for the experience. I knew I would lose, but I also knew women had entered more than once just for the experience and then later won. I planned to enter again when I was a senior at OCU.

My sorority friends were not just proud for me individually, they realized that any success I had brought favorable light on the sorority. They were my biggest fan club and always screamed and yelled at any event in which I participated. Cindy and Janis were cheerleaders at OCU, and knew how to scream and yell, and motivate a crowd.

Of course, we loved OCU basketball, led by legendary coach Abe Lemons, and spent many hours watching the beautiful Gary Gray on the court, as well as those great players from Rocky, Oklahoma, that Coach Lemons recruited. Another new friendship I made during my sophomore year was Beverly Drew, from Harrah, Oklahoma. She was my little sister in the sorority and a fellow music major.

For my talent in the Miss Oklahoma City pageant, I selected a medley from the musical "On a Clear Day You Can See Forever." Don Johnson helped me arrange the song and accompanied me. There were so many contestants and so many preliminaries. I did something really stupid before the swimsuit competition. Instead of shaving my legs, I tried depilatory cream. A bright red rash appeared without hours, so my legs were pink during the swimsuit competition in the preliminaries.

During the long wait in the preliminary competition, I became extremely nervous. I began clearing my throat, in fear that I would have a frog in my throat or be hoarse during my singing performance. I found out later that a sure way to become hoarse is to walk around constantly clearing your throat.

Apparently, hoarse voices and pink legs were in, because I made the top ten. In the evening gown competition, I wore the same $50 green dress my parents had made my Christmas present the year before. From the 22 contestants, I was fortunate to be among the 12 finalists chosen. The other finalists were Ginny Stevens, Sherry Parker, Nancy Childers, Patricia Gayle Polansky, Nancy Fisher, Lynda Martin, Karlene Alt, Mary Ann O'Connell, Jan Lawhon, Susan Sanderson, and Glenda Locust.

For the finals in the ballroom of the Sheraton-Oklahoma Hotel, pageant officials suggested all contestants wear a white evening gown. But I could not ask my parents to buy another dress, so I wore my old standby green dress. When I walked onto the stage, my parents probably wished I had asked them for extra money for a new dress. I really stood out as the only girl wearing anything but white.

Frankly, wearing the green dress may have been a plus for me. Clara

Luper, the legendary civil rights leader and educator in Oklahoma City, loves to tell the story of how she and her entourage pulled for me to win because she knew I had to feel self conscious about being the only girl in a colored dress.

I was the most surprised girl in the audience on April 28, 1966, when it was announced I was the new Miss Oklahoma City. Television personality Gaylon Stacy, the master of ceremonies, asked me for a comment, and I replied, "I'm a little too shook to say anything. I would like to say thank you to so many people-especially my friends at OCU."

I was handed the crown from the reigning Miss Oklahoma City, Kerry Williams, who later became one of my best friends for life. In addition to her career as an actress, Kerry became a huge television personality in Oklahoma City appearing with Danny Williams on "Dannysday" on WKY-TV.

The "shook" comment made its way into print in *The Daily Oklahoman* the following morning with the headline, "Miss Oklahoma City 'Shook.'" Reporter Mary Goddard described me as an OCU beauty with burnished brown hair and a lilting voice. She also pointed out that "unlike most of the white-clad contestants, Miss Jayroe appeared with her five feet, five inches and 116 pounds delectably distributed in an emerald green gown." I don't think I ever weighted 116 pounds, but it sounded good. I always felt "too big."

The runners-up for Miss Oklahoma City were Jan Lawhon, a freshman at the University of Oklahoma, and Ginny Stevens, a senior at OCU and Surrey Singer. Harry Schwartz was president of the Miss Oklahoma City Pageant and Curt, his son, was on the board. Curt became a wonderful friend.

As Miss Oklahoma City, I was entitled to move on to the Miss Oklahoma pageant. My hopes of performing and winning pageants were alive and well. However, my goal was to somehow convince OCU music officials to allow me to sing with the Surrey Singers, have many performing opportunities, and someday later, when I was older, enter the Miss America pageant.

I was only 19 and had no idea that "someday later" would come much sooner than I ever dreamed.

BEVERLY HOSTER

~ ~ ~ *"During our pageant years Jane was supremely successful. But her success did not stop her from encouraging me. I lost my first attempt at Miss Oklahoma. Shortly thereafter, I received a letter from Jane while she was busy in New York being Miss America. She encouraged me to try again. The next year Jane worked with me to improve my talent. This time I won and Jane was even happier than I was."*

TOM MCDANIEL

~ ~ ~ *"Jane symbolizes all that Oklahoma City University seeks to produce in a servant leader. A small-town Oklahoma girl, with big-league talent and world-class grace, she became Miss Oklahoma and Miss America while a student on our campus in 1967. Now, almost four decades later, she has returned to serve as the National Spokesperson for our Centennial and as director of special events for the university.*

Jane's beauty and poise provided her with extraordinary opportunities, and her commitment to her faith, her family, and her values helped her capitalize on them. She proved in 1967 that she was one of a kind. She still is!"

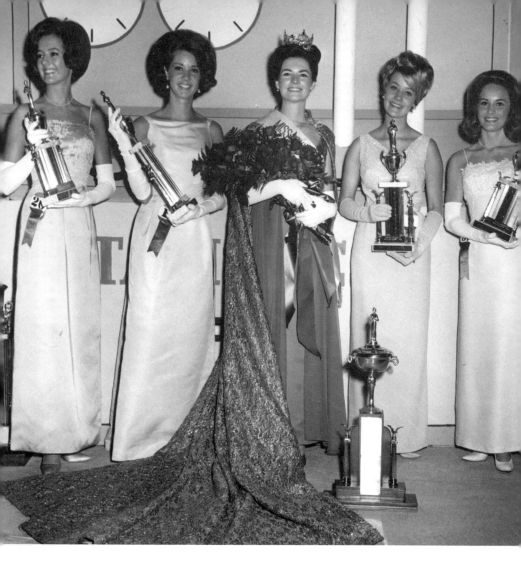

The top five finishers in the Miss Oklahoma Pageant in 1966. Left to right, Connie Criswell, Miss Northeastern State College, Sandy Ferguson, Miss Lawton, me, Carol Rich, Miss Duncan, and Lana Boyd, Miss Village.

6

MISS OKLAHOMA

Even though I had won the title of Miss Oklahoma City, I still was shy and insecure about being a beauty queen. A few days after winning the crown, arrangements were made for me to meet Debbie Bryant, Miss America 1966, during her visit to Oklahoma. I felt so out of place that I failed to show up for the meeting. I got all dressed up, drove around Jackie Cooper Oldsmobile's showroom a couple of times, and drove back home. I was such a ninny!

I had little time to consider the gravity of my entry in the Miss Oklahoma pageant that was scheduled in Tulsa less than two months after I won the crown as Miss Oklahoma City. I was busy trying to finish my semester of class work and directing my sorority sisters in a medley of tunes from the popular Broadway show *The Fantasticks*. We took first place in the women's division of the 19th annual May Day Sing at OCU. I was thrilled for my sisters.

With everything else going on, my schedule became incredibly heavy. I was given a wardrobe by Rothschilds Department Store as Miss Oklahoma City, although I wanted to make my own dress to use in the talent portion of the Miss Oklahoma pageant.

Donna House was so helpful in getting me prepared for the Miss Oklahoma pageant. She helped me with clothing and agreed with my decision to change my talent to a medley of "Your Love Makes Me Beautiful" and "Sadie, Sadie, Married Lady," from the musical *Funny Girl*.

My OCU family did everything they could to assure my success. Mrs.

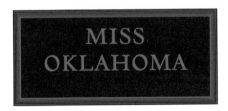

Apgar helped me with the music and played for me any time I felt like practicing. Mrs. Silberg also carefully listened to my singing and coached me to a new level of performance.

At the last minute, I decided that my talent costume was not what I wanted to wear, so Donna House loaned me a black outfit with fringe from her closet. Even though the Miss Oklahoma City sponsors were supportive, I do not think they expected me to win the Miss Oklahoma crown.

In early June, 1966, mother and I drove to Tulsa. It was the first time either of us had ever been to Tulsa and we were lost for awhile before we found the Mayo Hotel. I will never forget walking into the lobby and seeing so many beautiful girls who I thought were surely more experienced and more sophisticated than me. They were all from big cities and big universities, or so I thought. Although I was representing the state's largest city, I was still a simple, small town girl from western Oklahoma.

The Miss Oklahoma pageant was big time. Toni Spencer, the director, had a huge heart and worked hard to make every contestant feel important. Toni's creative flare and organizational skills made her superhuman. Toni was working in a world that emphasized beauty and physical perfection, even though she suffered from twisted hands and feet, the result of crippling arthritis that had stricken her in her twenties. Her handicap did not slow her a bit. In fact, there was something special about those crooked fingers waving directions, correcting a script, or buttoning a glove.

As usual, I committed to do my best, but I knew I would not win. Earlier, I had auditioned for Lyric Theater, been accepted for the chorus, and had made arrangements to live in an apartment with a friend for the summer in Oklahoma. There was no chance I would win the Miss Oklahoma title on the first try!

The talent competition was the first stage of the pageant. It counted 50 percent of the total score and there is so much that can go wrong. Your voice can break, you can trip, the microphone can go dead, you can forget your words, and the orchestra can mess up. Sandy Ferguson, a talented tap dancer from Lawton, Oklahoma, won the talent competition. She had a lot of help from great pageant supporters Bobbie and Don Glasby from Lawton.

The next day, I won the swimsuit preliminary; an area of competition that I felt was my weakest. Parading around in a swimsuit on stage is enough to give anyone goose bumps, shaky knees, the hiccoughs, a rash, or a muscle twitch, all of which has happened to me at one time or another during beauty pageant competitions.

The final test was the interview with the judges. I do not remember a thing I said. I had no idea if I had done well enough to qualify. For the finals, all I wanted to do was to finish in the top ten. At 3:00 p.m. in the afternoon of the finals, I began to feel dizzy and faint. I did not return to normal until the top ten girls were announced. I had made it. I could relax.

On Saturday night, June 11, I was at home on stage, performing the medley I had sung at least 2,000 times, even in my sleep. Somehow, I was named Miss Oklahoma. Not too many of my family members or friends from Laverne were in the audience because it was in the middle of wheat harvest season. However, several of my friends from OCU were in attendance. A picture in state newspapers showed me in shock, with my gloved hands over my face.

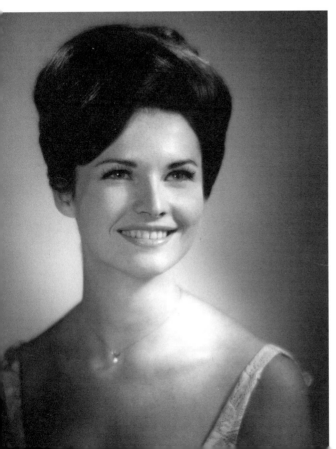

This official Miss Oklahoma photograph was included in all press packets that were handed out when I made an official visit.

There is an interesting story about me passing the crown of Miss Oklahoma City to the first runner up. I had to relinquish the crown because I was now Miss Oklahoma. At first, the title went to Jan Lawhon. Later, officials realized they had misread the rules and eliminated the first runner up, Ginny Stevens, by mistake. Ginny had married Don Johnson. In July, we gathered at the National Cowboy Hall of Fame and Western Heritage Center in Oklahoma City to rectify the situation.

With Oklahoma City Mayor George Shirk present, Jan gave the crown back to me, and I officially crowned Ginny. Then Ginny formally announced her wedding plans, resigned her crown, and passed it back to Jan. A newspaper reporter wrote, "Everybody was happy, although a bit confused."

To be Miss Oklahoma was my most fun win ever. I love Oklahoma very much and being Miss Oklahoma was a big deal. I received a lot of scholarship money to be able finish school. I was allowed to drive a brand new Oldsmobile, usually from Jackie Cooper. I did not have a car when I began school at OCU. Later I was given my parents' second car, a little red Ford Falcon in terrible shape. The new convertible had a sign on the side of the door, "Jayne Jayroe, Miss Oklahoma." I drove the car with great pride.

As I began to enjoy being Miss Oklahoma, it began to dawn on me that I had to compete in the Miss America pageant. Even though my whole life had been filled with dreams of doing so, every time I thought of going to Atlantic City, my palms would get moist and my stomach would be tied in knots. The only consolation was—there really was no way I could win this one.

KERRY ROBERTSON KERBY

~ ~ ~ *"Jane and I were friends long before either of us entered the world of television. We first met when I turned over my crown as Miss Oklahoma City to the new winner—Jane. After her reign as Miss America, we both married and became close friends with dreams about the future. Some of them came true, some of them did not. For many years, Jane has been a valued advisor, encourager, mentor, and most importantly a very generous and a dear friend. During many of our long walk and talks we have laughed and cried as we share the ups and downs of our lives. If the old saying, 'Friends are the jewels in your crown,' is true, Jane's crown is full of precious gems. Her friends are many long lasting—and there is a reason for that. Very simply, she is authentic, the real thing. In addition to all her great accomplishments and honors, Jane is still that down-to-earth girl from Laverne who loves the Lord, her family, her friends, and the state that has given her so many wonderful opportunities to shine."*

SUE WELLS

~ ~ ~ *"Janie and I were both from small town Oklahoma, she from the west, and me from the east. We were instant friends. She was an absolute luminous being of light and beauty—such a pure soul and profound role model. Janie was always an inspiration to me and others. Our lives touched at OCU and have been intertwined ever since. I believed the old adage, you can't choose your family, but you can choose your friends. I chose Janie for both. Since I was raised in an orphanage, I had room for both a family member and friend. Janie has always been there for me. Isn't that what a family is?"*

I was proud to represent my home state.

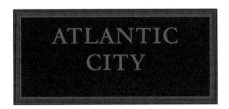

7

ATLANTIC CITY

had chosen to sing in the talent competition in both the Miss Oklahoma City and Miss Oklahoma pageants. However, Toni Spencer realized that for me to have any chance of winning in Atlantic City, my talent selection needed to be unique. After she discovered my love of musical conducting, she came up with the idea of me not only singing, but dancing and directing the orchestra.

Toni chose the great popular song "1,2,3" and rewrote some of the lyrics to bring in different sections of the orchestra in an effective way. It was a dynamite arrangement that was destined to make people smile and tap their toes. With the help of my sister, I determined how to perform to the music and then practiced singing, dancing, and directing an invisible orchestra at least 1,000 times. Mother's extension cord was my microphone, our garage was my stage, and our only tape recorder was the orchestra.

Mo Billingsley, who had conducted the orchestra in the Miss Oklahoma pageant, became my musical director and gave me a lot of advice. It was the ultimate performing challenge, but I would never have a chance to practice with a live band, on a stage, or with a sound system, until a one-time, five-minute rehearsal in Atlantic City. I wore the demo tape of the arrangement slick in the weeks before the pageant.

I was not a total music novice, but I felt very inadequate to direct an orchestra before a live television audience. In addition to 10 years of piano lessons, singing and performing in high school in college, I was also a music major and had taken classes in conducting from Dr. Ray Luke, a nationally recognized teacher and composer. But none of my past training seemed adequate. It was just the day-after-day rehearsal in the garage of our rented frame house in the summer heat of western Oklahoma.

Looking back, I am amazed at my own willingness to risk. Growing up in an environment that gave me so many opportunities may be responsible for that courage. I had stepped up to so many free throw lines under pressure, stood in front of judges at a music contest, and sang without warming up at church, and always went on to the next thing. In Atlantic City, I rehearsed my talent two times and it was the only time I performed it live before the pageant competition.

Toni kept in touch with me. She was a realist and actually prepared me to lose. And yet, I was determined to do my best and that was always my prayer. I never prayed to win. Toni would say, "Miss America is really hard work…and worse. It messes up a lot of people." In my heart I knew she was making certain I would not be disappointed emotionally by not winning. Oklahoma had not had a winner since Norma Smallwood in 1924, a third of a century before. Toni and I both knew that the 1966 entry, me, would not change that. I was prepared to lose. Winning was out of the realm of my thinking. Winning the Miss America crown happened to perfect people and even in my most confident moments I was not even close to perfect.

Toni spent much of her time working with my posture and teaching me how to talk. She conducted mock interviews with every conceivable question that might be asked me by the judges. She picked out all my clothing. My evening gown that Toni spent so much time selecting did not arrive at the store in time so I ended up with a substitute gown from Clark's Good Clothes in Tulsa.

Toni, in her desire to make me stand out among the other contestants was creative in getting me enrolled as an official Miss America contestant. Without her innovative talent idea, I would have been very fortunate to make the top ten. However, I was frankly a little uncomfortable with some of the information she put on my paperwork. She gave me a nickname, "Jay-Jay," which unfortunately stuck after I won. My name had been Janie growing up, and Jane in college, and my family and closest friends thought I was crazy when newspapers began saying my nickname was Jay-Jay.

Also, Toni put on the entry forms that I wanted to be a musical conductor of orchestras. That was not exactly the truth. I wanted to be a musical theater performer, although I was majoring in music education, which certainly contained a component of conducting.

By the middle of the summer my parents began talking about how we were going to get to Atlantic City. I had never flown in an airplane and did not think I wanted to start then. Plus, there was the expense of my parents. Toni knew that my dream had always been to see New York City and Broadway, so she planned a driving trip to New York before we were schedule to arrive for the Miss America competition in Atlantic City.

At the last minute, Toni announced she would not be able to go to New York and Atlantic City with me. I was devastated but understood what a toll Toni's absolute devotion to me as Miss Oklahoma had taken on her family. I had lived with her, her husband, and four children for days at a time.

Toni had big dreams for me. She even thought about publicity for me along the route from Laverne to New York City. At hotels along the way, she arranged to have me announced on the marquee. My parents and I began the long drive and were shocked when we drove up to a motel and saw a very visible sign, "Best Western welcomes Miss Oklahoma, Jayne Jayroe." Toni thought of everything. Our car was packed with all my gowns and hats. There was barely enough room for mother and me in the back seat.

New York City was better than I had dreamed. I took pictures at every corner, of taxis, street signs, and the incredible variety of people. We saw "Mame" with Angela Lansbury and "Sweet Charity" with Gwen Verden. I was smitten with Broadway. I treasured every moment in this huge city with gigantic billboards announcing the latest musicals because I knew that in less than two weeks I would be going back to Oklahoma and probably never get to see Broadway again. No where in my wildest imagination was an illusion that I could actually be Miss America and live in New York for the coming year.

It was finally time for us to drive to Atlantic City. Daddy got out the maps and plotted our trip into New Jersey. Atlantic City was unlike any city I had ever seen. The Boardwalk was unique. I learned that it was built over the beaches because hotels and elegant restaurants that had constructed along the shore hated the constant flow of sand into train cars and hotel lobbies. Construction of the boardwalk had begun in 1870, nearly a century before the Jayroes from Laverne had walked on its planks for the first time.

Atlantic City has a fabulous history of being "the place to go" on the eastern seaboard of the United States. It had become a world famous resort, home of the Miss America pageant, and the city that gave the world many "firsts"—the first airport, first saltwater taffy, first boardwalk, first postcards, and first use of the golf term "birdie."

I was not really nervous because I believed I had no chance of winning. What was there to be nervous about? When my mother and I walked into the initial reception for the contestants, I turned to her and said, "This is the last time I am going to do something like this."

Having to promote myself to strangers was painful. I was very shy and miserable when I had to tell people I had never seen before about my talent and why I deserved to be Miss America. It just was not my thing!

However, once we got into rehearsals, I was at home. I loved the time with the other girls. I made friends and enjoyed the actual competition. The judges interview session with two other contestants and me went amazingly well. What served me best was my inner peace that I had done all I could to prepare, I was who I was, and not a likely winner, and that I was grateful to be living my dream. I was just so happy to be in Atlantic City, to be part of this competition.

In the preliminary interview process, I was paired with one of the other contestants, Barbara Ann Harris, Miss South Carolina. She had a lot of pressure on her to win the competition. I had none. She was her state's best entry in years and appeared to be perfect—a wonderful operatic voice, a gorgeous body, a soft southern voice, and sparkling blue eyes and dimples.

I was in awe of the judges, Vincent Price, the deep-voiced actor, conductor Donald Voorhees, and Onna White, who had choreographed "Mame" that I had just seen on Broadway. I was honored to meet them and Skip Henderson, the famous musical conductor. When they asked me questions, I was cool and calm, trying to sincerely express my delight at being there with them. When someone asked me a serious question about conducting, I quipped, "You know, I just want to keep time to the music!" Skip Henderson thought that answer was hysterical.

In comparison to my answers, Barbara Ann stumbled under the pressure of a serious question about the racial situation in the South. She was nervous and her answer came out opposite of what she intended. She knew it, but the more she tried, the worse it got. I genuinely felt compassion for her.

The pace was frantic during rehearsals. The all day rehearsals ruined my feet that already were in bad shape. I have flat feet and standing in high heels and pageant shoes made my feet hurt badly. My mother was so supportive—when I arrived at the hotel room at night after rehearsal, she had a hot bath ready for me. I soaked my feet for what seemed like hours.

On Friday night, I performed for the judges on the Miss America stage that seemed to be as long as football field. I loved being Miss Oklahoma on that stage. I had worked for years to get to this point, but was still prepared to lose. The highest place I could ever imagine was runner up. After all, Toni had told me about Anita Bryant, the Oklahoma girl who had been runner up and parlayed the second place finish into great career opportunities.

In the back of my mind, I was thinking about missing the first two weeks of classes at OCU. I had moved into the dormitory with my roommate. OCU had been completely accommodating about me missing classes, but I was still a little apprehensive about having to catch up. And, there was my responsibility as Miss Oklahoma. There were at least a dozen appearances already scheduled for the few months before Christmas.

Only my parents were in the audience for the talent competition on Friday night. My sister, Judy, was teaching in Pampa, Texas. Money was just too scarce in our family to be able to bring her to the pageant. My father jokingly told one of the other fathers in Atlantic City that he could not afford for his daughter to win any more honors. It was an expensive effort for my family. Aunt Honore and cousin, Mary, were planning to come in for the final night of the pageant, but only my mother and father were present when the judges announced that I had won the talent competition.

I was shocked. I had listened to so many impressive voices and watched very talented girls dance better than I had ever seen. How could I be the talent winner? I thought, "This must be a fluke!" Even with the talent win behind me, I continued to trust my judgment that there was no way I could be Miss America. However, it made me think twice about the possibility of finishing in the top ten.

I was very self conscious in the swim suit competition. I had to stand next to Barbara Ann, Miss South Carolina. Our measurements were listed as the same, but we were not even close. Fudging on such statistics was standard in beauty pageants. She was tiny and I felt like a big basketball player standing next to her.

The real front runner in the pageant was Miss California, Charlene Diane Dallas, who won the preliminary swimsuit and talent competition and turned out to be first runner up in the entire pageant. She was stunningly beautiful and played classical piano. She had a whole entourage of people with her. All the girls had heard about her $1,000 evening gown. The buzz was that surely Charlene would win—her name even sounded like a Miss America. Even the newspapers believed Charlene would win. The *Philadelphia Bulletin,* on the morning of the final competition, reported that Charlene had won the swimsuit competition and called her the "favorite" for the Miss America title.

My dream was realized when it was announced that I had made the top ten. That meant that I would appear on national television—my recurrent dream since I had snuggled close to the television as a small girl while beautiful girls sang and danced and the lucky one walked the 120-foot runway at Convention Hall in Atlantic City.

I was so honored to perform my talent selection on television. I was promoting the great state that had given me so much. I was dressed in black tights with a tie and tails and boldly stepped to the orchestra pit, took the baton from Glen Osser, and led the orchestra in a swinging novelty version of "1, 2, 3."

I continued to keep my wits about me. My top ten finish had been accomplished and I still knew I had no chance of winning. My nerves were calm even when I made the top five and joined Miss California, Charlene Dallas; Miss Tennessee, Vicki Lynn Hurd; Miss Ohio, Sharon Elaine Philliam; and Miss New Hampshire, Nancy Anne Naylor, on the stage to appear for questions from Bert Parks, the magnificent veteran host of the pageant.

I certainly did not expect the question, "Do you expect to encounter prejudice in your desire to become a musical conductor?" First of all, it was only a half-truth, Toni's idea, that I wanted to conduct. So, I answered, "I know that I will run into prejudice. But I am studying not only to conduct and learn to become a conductor, but I want to learn about voice and piano and music generally." I also said, "I think that if you're talented enough,

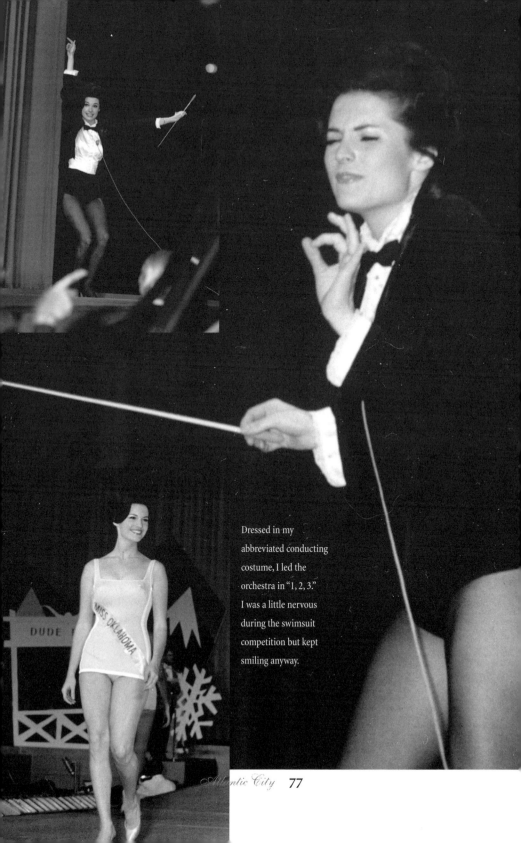

Dressed in my abbreviated conducting costume, I led the orchestra in "1, 2, 3." I was a little nervous during the swimsuit competition but kept smiling anyway.

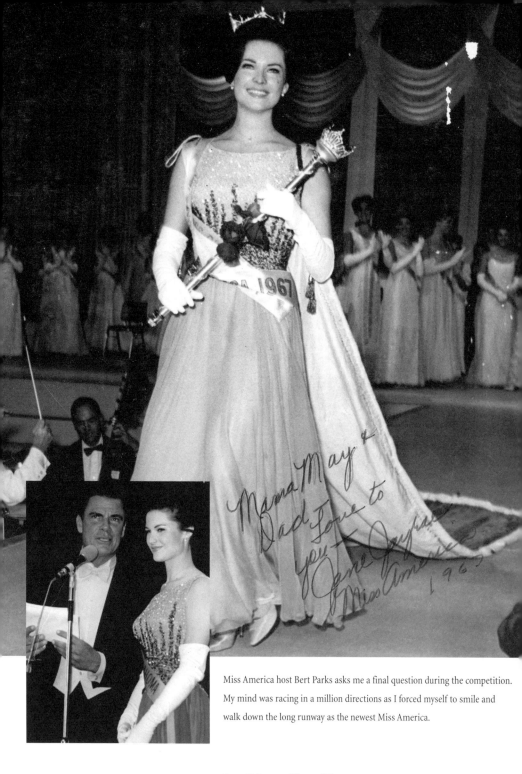

*Mama May &
Dad — Love to
you
Jane Jayroe
Miss America
1967*

Miss America host Bert Parks asks me a final question during the competition.
My mind was racing in a million directions as I forced myself to smile and
walk down the long runway as the newest Miss America.

there will be a way for you to attain it." I still look back at that answer and realize how immature I was at 19 and how I had no idea how to answer that question. If I did not have a compulsion to be truthful, it would have been easier to answer. I did love conducting, but I also knew I was more performer than musical director.

When the judging got down to just Miss California and me, I was still okay with the fact that I now had won the coveted first runner up spot. I did not worry about it, especially when Bert walked in front of Charlene and me and I saw "Miss California" written on the piece of paper in his hand. That told me Charlene had won—I did not for a moment realize that what was written on the paper was the name of the runner up.

My court and me backstage after I won the Miss America crown. Left to right, Miss Ohio, Sharon Elaine Philliam, Miss California, Charlene Diane Dallas, Miss Tennessee, Vicki Lynn Hurd, Miss New Hampshire, Nancy Ann Naylor, and me.

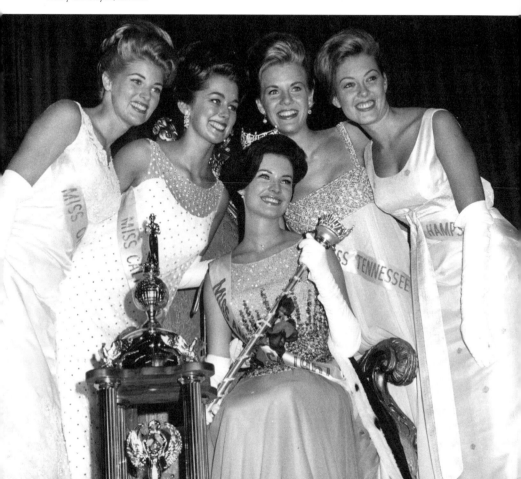

Shock is an understatement of what I felt when Charlene was announced first runner up. My mind was racing—wait a minute, that means I won! It was impossible—Charlene, Barbara Ann, so many other girls were more talented and more glamorous than me.

The more than 20,000 people in the Convention Hall roared to their feet. Flash bulbs blinded me as I was handed a huge bouquet of roses and the Miss America crown was placed on my head by the outgoing Miss America, Deborah Bryant from Kansas. As Bert sang, "There She is, Miss America," I walked down that long runway to an endless roar of applause. I was so stunned I could hardly breathe. I was not supposed to win. I was planning to drive back to Oklahoma the next day and move into the dormitory at OCU.

I was totally unaware that massive television cameras were recording my every move down the runway—that all my friends, family, and teachers, and members of my church in Laverne, and my OCU friends in Oklahoma City were all gathered around television sets. Anyone who had a color set had a houseful of visitors that night.

I told myself not to cry—but my brain did not listen. Tears streamed down my face. Then my walk down the runway was over. I ascended a golden staircase on the stage and stood before my throne wiping tears with my white elbow-length gloves. Then, it hit me like a ton of bricks—I was Miss America.

BILL THRASH

~ ~ ~ *"I was at KOCO-TV on the Saturday night when the Associated Press wire flashed the new Miss America was from Oklahoma. It was 9:55 p.m. But the NBC Miss America telecast was a one-hour delay, so few people knew the outcome. In the commercial television competitive spirit, I had our anchor lead with the story that the new Miss America was from Laverne.*

What I failed to realize was that the vast majority of Oklahomans were watching the pageant on NBC and our great scoop went largely unnoticed." ~

RON NORICK

~ ~ ~ *"Jane is an exciting ambassador for Oklahoma. Whether in public life or as a private citizen, she promotes the great qualities of our state."*

MELVIN MORAN

~ ~ ~ *"I met Jane a few months after she was crowned Miss America. My wife, Jasmine, and I directed the Miss Seminole pageant and Jane accepted our invitation to attend the event. On the date of the pageant, Jane arrived in Seminole and fulfilled her promise to attend a tea/reception. Following that event, I told Jane that it was not on her schedule but another organization wondered if she could something with them. She said, "Yes, of course." The day stretched into a dozen appearances. Jane could not have been more gracious and said yes every time we asked her. She did not get a moment's rest for a 12-hour period from the time she arrived in Seminole until the end of the pageant. "*

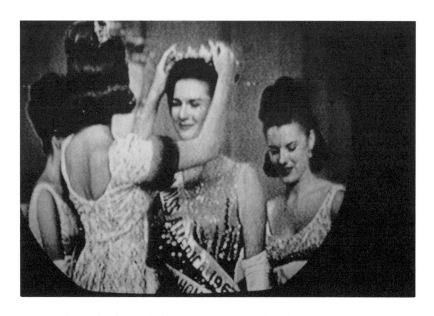

A fan sent this photograph of the crowning as it appeared on television.

8

A SHAKY START

After the curtain closed, I was ushered backstage to receive the congratulations of the other contestants and to begin the unending posing for photographs. I was no longer an unknown girl from western Oklahoma who had been blessed to win the Miss Oklahoma title. I was now a celebrity—and the first moments gave me a bad feeling that I had a tough year ahead of me.

It was like being one of the Beatles—I could not move backstage without security people keeping others away from me. Somehow, members of the audience had slipped backstage. One girl was screaming my name and desperately trying to touch my gown. The shock of winning quickly grew into fear of what winning meant. Policemen were everywhere. No one could get to me—and I could not find my parents—they were lost in the crowd. It was pandemonium.

I was one scared little girl when police escorted me out of Convention Hall toward a waiting car. I spent the night in my hotel room with the head of hostesses for the pageant, a lady I had just met. She just glared at me while I sobbed. She must have thought, "What a stupid, stupid girl!" It would have helped me that night if someone could have just consoled me with simple words such as, "Hey, Janie, we're going to take care of you. Don't worry. Some really nice things are going to happen to you." My mother was my chaperone and was with me, but she did not know anything either, except that she would be sent home on Monday and leave me—with whom? I cried all night.

In between patches of sleep I thought of what was happening to me. No one has ever believed me that I did not want to be Miss America at that time. It was like I got ahead of myself. I know that sounds horrible, but I was so immature and unprepared for such a role. I was 19 and wanted to be with my friends and audition for the chorus in summer theater. I wanted to go home to Laverne and feel like I belonged. As Miss America, I had agreed not to date for a year, to be told what to wear, where to go, and what to say. I did not want to travel every day and continuously be with strangers who would sit and stare at me for hours. I wanted to giggle, be sloppy, have fun, and be me—Janie Jayroe—not Miss America. Yikes!

If Bert Parks had asked me what I wanted to be in 10, 15, or 20 years, I would have probably answered, "I want to be married, have children, teach school, do a lot of rewarding volunteer work, and live happily ever after." But, my life was on hold. I was committed to living out of a suitcase and "serving" an entire year as Miss America. I had no idea what that meant, other than I could not have my mother with me. I was terrified.

What did I know about being Miss America? All I had been told about the year ahead was contained in a six-page letter that was waiting in my hotel room. The letter, addressed generically to "Miss America 1967," was from Lenora Slaughter, the executive director of the pageant who had over-seen 32 pageants. Lenora was so right when she said, "You are going to have many conflicting emotions as you try to set your house in order...To say you are confused is putting it mildly. But through the confusion will contin-ue to ring the "bell of happiness, success, and anticipation." At the moment, that bell had not yet begun to ring.

Sunrise in Atlantic City helped my feelings. My handlers briefed me on what would be a whirlwind day. I finally grasped the extent of the monetary awards that accompany the Miss America title. I was given a $10,000 college scholarship and promised $75,000 in appearance fees. To collect the fees for appearing at all kinds of places in every state of the union, I pledged to trav-el more than 200,000 miles.

My first appointment of the morning was in a photograph session with *Life* magazine. Then, I held my first press conference. What did I know about press conferences? The most I had ever talked to a reporter was back stage after winning the Miss Oklahoma pageant. Now, dozens of print reporters and several television camera crews camped out beyond the bank of microphones which were placed before me.

After a few questions, I was reasonably comfortable talking to the reporters. I told them, "I thought only polished ladies from big cities won the title of Miss America." I told them about me wanting to be a fourth generation school teacher and about my mother, father, and sister being involved in education. I also said I hoped to be able to go to Vietnam to entertain American soldiers who were so far away from home. Throughout the year, the press was amazingly kind to me. They never once expected me to have the answer to world peace.

I attended a luncheon with state queens, pageant directors, and Miss America officials. I felt so isolated and alone. Even though I was inundated with telegrams, flowers, and phone calls, I was truly shaken. "How wonderful," I thought, "that these people are so happy for me. Why am I so unhappy?"

God allowed a strange event, no doubt an example of His grace, to happen after the luncheon. I was not supposed to receive any phone calls in my room while I freshened up. But the telephone rang and I picked it up. It was a warm voice form my past that reached out in grace to give me peace for the moment and courage for the future.

It was Reverend Leonard Gillingham, my favorite minister when I was growing up. Leonard, as he insisted upon being called, was such an effective servant of the Lord. He was the only person who could convince my father to go to church with mother, Judy, and me. It was Leonard who had baptized Daddy and me on a glorious Sunday evening in Sentinel when I was 12.

To this day, I do not remember any part of the actual conversation with Leonard, but what I experienced was grace. My internal trauma subsided somewhat because I knew that when my parents left me in a few hours to return home, I would not be alone in New Jersey, New York, or any other place on earth. I was reminded in such a powerful way of the Apostle Paul's words from Philippians 4:13, "I can do all things through Christ who strengthens me." Whether I was a success or failure for the next 365 days was not up to me alone. I had the ultimate friend, God. I did not have to be everything to everybody. My childhood teaching came through loud and clear. It was enough for the moment just to belong to God and experience His power and grace. Even though I was not prepared on the external for this big role, God had been preparing me internally for years if only I would trust Him.

I was still shaky, especially when I thought of my parents driving away and leaving me in New Jersey. The final event of my first day as Miss America was a formal dinner with national pageant officials. I only knew them by name and was aware that they had opposed me actually conducting the orchestra as part of my talent performance. Later the Miss America pageant officially prohibited orchestra conducting.

It was a small group at dinner. They certainly did not seem thrilled that I had won—and I did not want to be there. Most of the participants at the dinner seemed to be the "partying" type. I am not a partier. I love to get to know people, but I was really uncomfortable with an environment of excessive drinking and sitting for hours at an extended meal.

I sat red-eyed, head down, just enjoying the company of my genuine, honest, and loving parents from Oklahoma. I was not trusting God fully, yet. How sad for me that I believed in my dream but did not trust God with the reality that I had won the Miss America crown. What if Sara in the Old Testament had balked when Abraham had said they had to leave everything because God had called him? What about Rebecca leaving her family and homeland? What about Ruth? The Bible is full of men and women who were called beyond themselves. In my frailty, I was not ready to receive God's grace and guidance. Years later, I read a book by Scott Peck and realized what my mental frame of mind had been. Peck wrote, "All of us are called by grace…but few of us choose to listen to the call." I certainly was hard of hearing.

Finally, the dinner conversation turned to my lackluster attitude. The business manager began lecturing me about how much money I was going to make and how appreciative I should be. My father stepped into the gap for me and quickly let him know that money was not the primary concern of our lives and that the Jayroe family was quite capable of surviving without anything the business manager had to offer. The business manager was all business—he told me that if I did not want to be Miss America, Miss California was more than ready to take my place.

At that moment, my sense of responsibility kicked in. Even though I was intimidated, scared, and horribly depressed at what I saw, I had to do what I was supposed to do. My parents had taught me that principle. I had been awarded one of the greatest honors on earth and I would be letting down the people of Oklahoma if I gave up my crown. I needed a sign from God that I could survive. It was like going away to camp for the first time. I was desperate for my mother not to leave, but if she did, I needed a warm substitute for the transition.

Into my life came Peg O'Neil—warm, bubbly, and a take charge kind of woman. She was retiring as a Miss America chaperone, but her long conversation with my parents after dinner made an incredible difference. I am not certain that my father would have left his little girl in Atlantic City and returned with mother to Oklahoma unless Peg assured him that I would be fine. Peg was a former teacher and completely related to my parents. Along with Bill Muncrief from Arkansas, Peg convinced my parents that being Miss America had little to do with the "partying" world and the people we had met at dinner.

In fairness to the pageant officials, it was a difficult time for them. The Miss America office was in a time of transition. Lenora Slaughter and her husband, Brad Frapart, who had made the pageant into a major American institution, were about to leave. Chaperone changes were being made. Peg was moving to the front office. Irene Bryant, my new chaperone, was not yet on the job. Nor was Lucille Preveti, who would eventually share chaperone responsibilities with Irene.

I also felt better when I spent some time that evening with my parents and sat and read the hundreds of telegrams, notes, and newspaper articles I had received. I was embarrassed at the Atlantic City newspapers analysis of why I had won:

Miss Oklahoma gained the favor of judges with a bouncy presentation which included a bit of a song, swinging dance patterns, and a routine, during which she conducted the large pageant orchestra in an alluring cut-away costume of a conductor…The costume was cut away to reveal her lovely limbs and she probably was the most attractive conductor to stand before an orchestra.

Even though the *Atlantic City Press* covered my selection of Miss America in spectacular fashion, I was most thrilled that my home state of Oklahoma was so proud.

The *Altus Times-Democrat* said that Oklahomans had been searching since statehood for a spirit of pride and unity. The newspaper said pleas such as "pride in Oklahoma" had created no significant excitement, but that my selection as Miss America had changed that. The Altus editor wrote, "But now. . . aw, now! Oklahomans are rolling out of the east side mountains and prancing from the west prairies in a spirit of all-for-one. The one we're all for, of course is a lovely young lady from a little town called Laverne. She is Jayne Jayroe, the new Miss America."

My hometown newspaper in Laverne had a large headline, "Jane Wins Crown," in type that was usually reserved for announcing the beginning of a war or the death of a president. The *Laverne Leader Tribune* said so many nice things like, "Jane has been Laverne's queen for a long time, so to many of her friends here the Atlantic City judges only reaffirmed what we already believed."

The *Leader Tribune* story also said, "Laverne residents could no longer contain themselves after the television show was completed and everybody knew the results. Phones rang off the walls…Cars began streaming down Main Street with lights shining and horns blaring. The town siren blew, and many got out their left over firecrackers and generally made a noisy time of it."

The Laverne newspaper also picked up on the fact that I had changed my name back to Jane, rather than Jayne. "When she was in high school here," the newspaper story said, "she wanted to change her name a little, so she made it Jayne. In the official Miss America Pageant program book is carried as Jane and that's what we're going to do unless Miss America herself tells us she has come other preference."

The state's largest newspaper, *The Daily Oklahoman,* under a headline, "Not a Dry Eye in the State," gave me tremendous coverage. Reporter Jim Rogers was at the Alpha Chi Omega corner of the Panhellenic House on the OCU campus and wrote that "mascara was wasted by the handful." Rogers said, "Fingernails were gnawed, hands were wrung, and no dry handkerchiefs were seen. Rogers reported that when I was announced as the winner,

"Gleeful laughs, whoops, sobs, pleads, well wishes, and other expressions drowned out the TV's sound."

The newspaper reported that residents of my dormitory, Banning Hall, knew before the delayed broadcast that I had won. House mother Elizabeth Jones had received a call from United Press International that conveyed the message, "Your girl has won!" However, most of the girls had abandoned the dormitory living room for other venues that had a color television.

I learned later that my boyfriend, Rick Schuerman, a junior from St. Louis, Missouri, did not escape the attention of his girlfriend becoming Miss America. He was tossed into the OCU Eternal Fountain by his proud fraternity brothers.

My father brought me newspapers from all over the country. He somehow had found a shop in the hotel that carried newspapers from major cities. My photograph wearing my crown was on the front page on so many newspapers. I was greatly humbled by the publicity.

The next day I was even further humbled when I learned that a baby girl born in Laverne two days after I became Miss America was named after me. Laverna Jane Martin, a bouncy, seven-pound, five-ounce girl, the daughter of an oil field driller and his wife who had moved to Laverne just six weeks before, was named for both Laverne and me.

As I began my first full work day as Miss America as a guest on the Mike Douglas television show, my fellow students at OCU were celebrating a day off from classes. The administration's official policy was against walkouts, but more than half of the school's 2,700 students abandoned classes and formed a procession that was several blocks in length as they marched around the campus. As the march caught on, the crowd began sporting signs, "Yea, Jayne, Our Miss America" and "We are so proud of you, Jane!" Students chanted, "Walk out for Jayne!" OCU officials were obviously very proud of me, and looked the other way. No one got in trouble for walking out and celebrating my instant celebrity status.

Mom Jones, our dormitory house mother, stood guard over my dorm room, Room 103, where I obviously would not be staying. She told a newspaper reporter, "She'll make a wonderful Miss America. There's just something about her—she has poise and dignity, but she can put on a pair of cut off jeans and a shirt and be a whole lot of fun."

After the appearance on the Mike Douglas Show with fellow guest, Minnie Pearl, I was shuttled to a fashion show in New York City. I had a prepared speech, but did not deliver it very well. I was wrapped in furs, jewelry, and pampering by Lola Martin Costigan of BanLon. She was one of the many angels who would grace my life in the weeks to come.

A scary year loomed in front of me. But I was determined to make it—one day at a time.

CONNIE THRASH MCGOODWIN

~ ~ ~ *"I estimate there are 1,200 women across America who if polled would list Jane as their friend, 380 who would say she was one of their "closest" friends, and at least 37 would list her as their "best" friend. It may be her Miss America training, but Jane has an incredible ability to make every person she talks to feel special. She loves young people and loves being a mentor and role model. Jane works harder at maintaining her friendships than anyone I know. She is always coming up with schemes and ideas from classes to Bible studies and trips so she can be with her friends. Jane and I have weekly "walk 'n talks" at which we practice "creative whining." Actually, it is a positive experience because we allow ourselves "venting" time but then we analyze the situation and try to figure out why we are being wronged. Eventually, we laugh, acknowledge how blessed we are, and move on."*

JANE PELLEY

~ ~ ~ *"As a nine-year-old, I watched Jane crowned as Miss America from the living room of my home in Mooreland, Oklahoma. Our paths crossed professionally when she was hired as news anchor at KXAS-TV in Fort Worth/Dallas. These were the years when beauty queens and beautiful men began to push into news anchor chairs across the country. I was an ambitious journalism student working behind the scenes and many of us were skeptical about the "talking heads" on the set. Jane proved the skeptics wrong. She was a hard worker who was gracious and determined. She became a terrific success at KXAS and used her talents and gifts wisely to build an impressive career."*

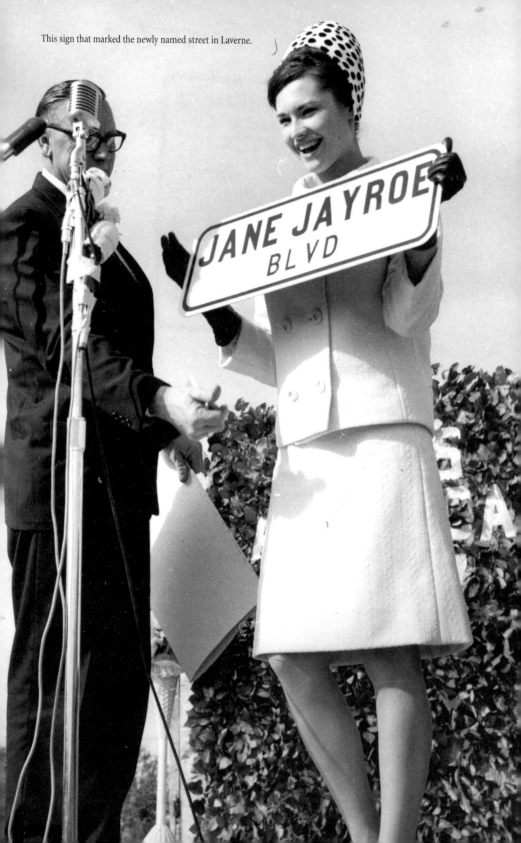

This sign that marked the newly named street in Laverne.

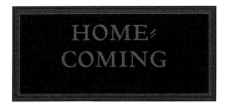

9

HOME COMING

*I*n the weeks following my crowning, I traveled to various cities in the United States. A lot of time was spent making appearances for the four national sponsors of the Miss America Pageant—Joseph Bancroft & Sons Company, the Pepsi-Cola Company, the Toni Company, and the Oldsmobile Division of General Motors. I had already received invitations to visit nine foreign countries, but pageant officials put those requests on hold.

Ban-Lon supplied me with many of my beautiful clothes from cocktail dresses to street clothes. I was told, "You can no longer dress as the typical school girl, for you will be constantly traveling and looked upon as a young woman who sets the standard in the world of American fashions." I learned to appreciate the Bancroft company representative, Lola Martin Costigan, who helped me dress in the latest and most attractive fashions.

Oldsmobile pledged to have a beautiful automobile awaiting me at every airport where I was making a public appearance. The Toni Company provided hairstylists and products to keep me looking "well groomed at all times." Toni marketed home permanents, so I was not allowed to wear any hair pieces. I was only allowed to drink Pepsi in public, although I certainly did not mind that rule.

Meanwhile, my beloved Oklahoma kept up the showering of praise. *The Daily Oklahoman* wrote on its editorial page, "Her natural grace and simplicity could have been the principal attribute that commended her to the judges. All Oklahoma takes pride in her."

I was really amazed at what appeared in the *Norman Transcript,* comparing me to my heroes. The newspaper article said, "Jayne Ann will add greatly to the national prestige of the stage which has been built up in the past by Will Rogers, the musical play *Oklahoma!,* and Bud Wilkinson's football teams at OU." I had never thought of myself anywhere near the league of Will Rogers and Bud Wilkinson.

The *Stillwater News-Press* recognized that being Miss America was being part of a commercial enterprise that might sell soap, shampoo, shoes, and "all sorts of goods which the Miss America image can profitably enhance." The article continued, "But that's all right, too. This is a commercial society, and we hope Miss Jayroe will help sell lots of soap, shampoo, and shoes to the mutual profit of us all."

I had to learn so much about being Miss America. I was given a stack of rules to learn. I was told not to make commitments to anyone, family, friends, well wishers, or the public, until I had time to make proper emotional adjustments. I was also told to feel free to express my opinion on world events, but only if I was sufficiently versed on the subject to "speak without embarrassment." I was not allowed to smoke or drink in public. I had no problems obeying that rule.

Other pieces of advice were to be humble and express a sincere desire to live up to the honor which had been bestowed upon me. Written comments from the executive director reminded me that the pageant office had to approve and schedule every day of the next year. In other words, my life, as the 39th Miss America, was their life.

The pageant office handled the business and personal side of my reign as Miss America. Phone calls were screened to sift the phonies from real invitations and offers. I was expected to be gracious, charming, and lovely at all times and to follow the instructions of my chaperones.

Each day was much the same. I arose early and dressed in a suit and hat. Miss America at that time was not allowed to wear slacks, and the hat was a must because the American Millinery Association provided hats to Miss America. I learned to fall asleep on airplanes before takeoff with an incredibly efficient system of removing my hat, putting my carry on luggage away, grabbing a blanket and pillow, and closing my eyes in less than one minute.

The travel was extensive—changing planes, sitting in airports, knitting, reading, changing to another plane. When we arrived, on went the hat, lipstick, and a Miss America smile for the awaiting crowd.

I was always the last person off the plane. There usually was a band playing and someone handed me a dozen roses. I signed autographs, said hello to everyone, and kept smiling. When I complained to my mother how I had begun to dislike arrivals, she gently reminded me that the people in the new city did not know I had been somewhere else yesterday and would be somewhere else tomorrow. They were simply excited about hosting Miss America.

I soon had appeared at more Oldsmobile showrooms and automobile shows that I knew existed. On most mornings in a new place, I stood in a small, roped-off area in a dealer's showroom or auto show, wearing my gown and crown. Soon I thought, "This is absurd—nobody goes around in an evening gown at 10:00 in the morning." However, on one occasion when I did not wear a gown, a little girl refused to give me roses because she said, "You can't be Miss America!" When asked why, she said Miss America should wear a crown and gown, not a suit and a hat. For hours, I would sit on a portable "throne" and hand out autographed post cards of me, and smile. I learned to smile and yawn at the same time. But if you looked closely, you could see my eyes watering.

It was hard to try to look like Miss America every day. I dealt constantly with meeting people whose faces showed disappointment when they thought Miss America was going to be such a knock out. Once when I had a fever, a child walked up for my autograph and shouted to her mother, "Look, Miss America has a cold sore!"

After a month on the road as Miss America, I was really getting homesick. I had not seen anyone from Oklahoma since I had won, not my sister, pageant director, or friends. The pageant office had scheduled three days in my native Oklahoma in late October. The days before I flew home dragged by slowly, although I was so busy from breakfast to dinner, crisscrossing America.

I did get one great gift on October 8. Miss America was booked by Oldsmobile for the Texas State Fair during the OU/Texas football weekend. Even though I did not get to see many of my friends, it was a chance to see my parents, Aunt Honore and her family, and some Oklahomans. I was featured early Saturday morning in a parade, then participated in a ribbon cutting for the opening of the Texas State Fair. Because of my connection to the football game, I was part of the halftime ceremony, which was a great surprise to the Oklahoma crowd.

When I appeared on the field sitting on the back of a convertible driven by my cousin's friend, Baker Montgomery, the crowd went wild. Baker stopped in from the OU band and I conducted them in "Oklahoma!" It was such a high, I thought surely I would fly out of the Cotton Bowl! From the

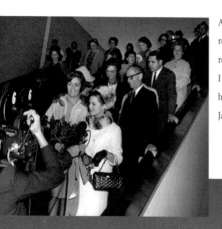

A dozen roses, pageant director Toni Spencer, and a score of reporters were on hand at Tulsa International Airport when I returned to Oklahoma for the first time. I was glad to be home! I have always been humbled by the attention given me by my hometown, especially the sign over Main Street that was renamed Jane Jayroe Boulevard.

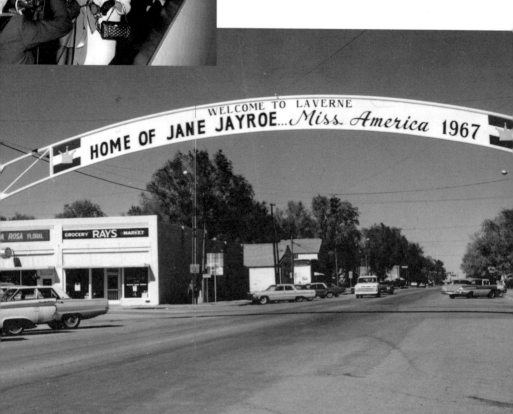

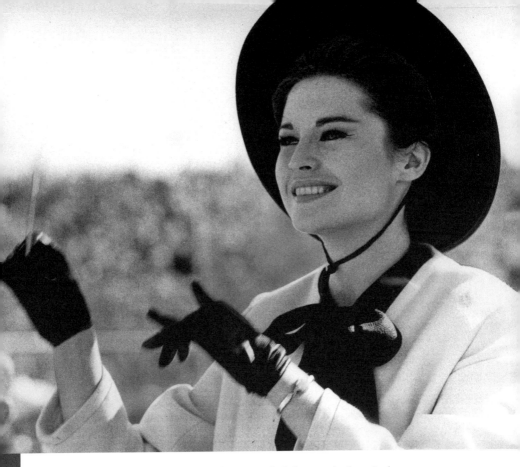

I was so happy to see people from Oklahoma at the OU-Texas football game at the Cotton Bowl. The fans cheered when I directed the OU band. Courtesy Oklahoma Publishing Company.

Oklahoma section, I rode in the car around to the Texas side and refused to give the "hook 'em horns" sign. I am sure I was not their favorite Miss America at that moment. OU beat Texas that year 18-9.

On October 20, 1967, I flew to Tulsa, Oklahoma. From the second I stepped off the plane, the excitement was intense. If the beginning of my time as Miss America was shaky because I was so overwhelmed, it was more real now and it was pure joy. Finally, the thrill of winning was shared with the people I loved. Toni Spencer and the Miss Oklahoma Pageant people met me at the airport. My parents were there. My sorority sisters were there.

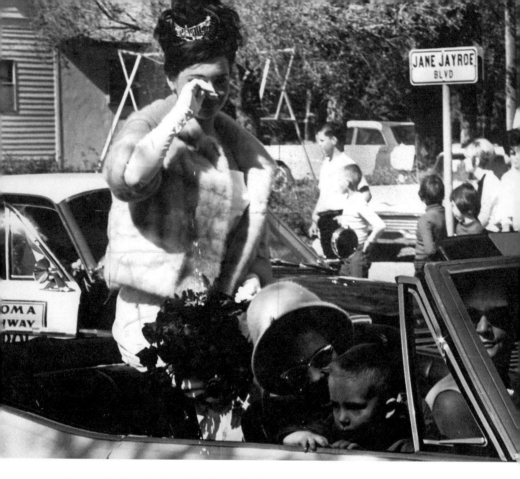

It was the beginning of a three-day joy ride with tears in my eyes and gratitude in my heart. At long last, I was home in Oklahoma and nothing could have been sweeter.

That evening I attended a reception for patrons of the Miss Oklahoma Pageant and appeared in a nighttime parade, complete with floats, clowns, and bands, through the streets of Tulsa. I felt like a princess riding through my kingdom. One of the parade promoters estimated the crowd at 40,000 to 50,000. I was perched on the back of a shining convertible. I was dressed in a sparkling green and gold gown and mink jacket.

It was windy and chilly, but people cheered and pushed so close to my car that we were forced to stop until a motorcycle escort could clear the way. One little boy had climbed to the top of a traffic light for a better view. I was overwhelmed and paid Tulsans the supreme compliment—I was moved to

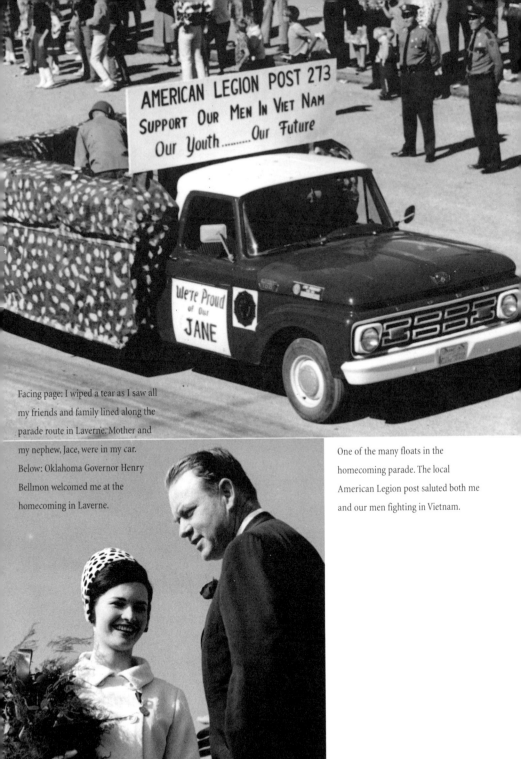

Facing page: I wiped a tear as I saw all my friends and family lined along the parade route in Laverne. Mother and my nephew, Jace, were in my car. Below: Oklahoma Governor Henry Bellmon welcomed me at the homecoming in Laverne.

One of the many floats in the homecoming parade. The local American Legion post saluted both me and our men fighting in Vietnam.

AMERICAN LEGION POST 273
SUPPORT OUR MEN IN VIET NAM
Our Youth.........Our Future

We're Proud of Our JANE

tears. The *Tulsa World* said it was a great parade, but that I was the star. Because I was home in Oklahoma, I really felt the love from my new 40,000 friends.

I could not wait to see the rest of my family and friends in Laverne as I boarded a private jet in Tulsa the following morning. We flew to Woodward and then drove in a motorcade to Laverne. Everybody in northwest Oklahoma knew about my homecoming because a motorcade of 20 cars carrying 140 high school band members and civic boosters had made a 486-mile tour of several cities and towns to publicize the Homecoming Day. My dad accompanied the caravan, although mother was unable to leave her classes. Booster tour director Cecil Mitchell's goal was to have 10,000 people present for my appearance.

When I arrived in town, it looked as if every man, woman, and child who lived within 50 miles were waiting for me. We drove down what was formerly Main Street—city fathers had recently named it Jane Jayroe Boulevard. What an honor! Laverne had such a pristine look about it. Buildings had been repainted, streets were re-graveled, and new street signs on "my" street gleamed in the morning sun.

The Friday edition of the *Enid Morning News* set the tone for the celebration with an editorial titled "It's Jane Ann's Homecoming."

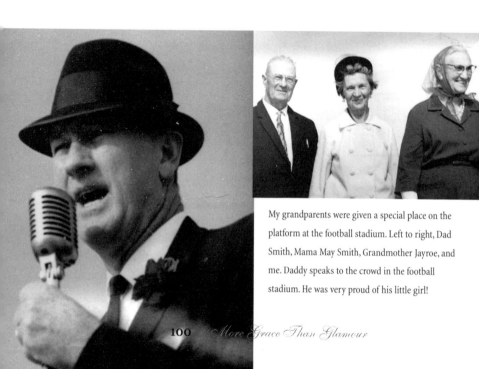

My grandparents were given a special place on the platform at the football stadium. Left to right, Dad Smith, Mama May Smith, Grandmother Jayroe, and me. Daddy speaks to the crowd in the football stadium. He was very proud of his little girl!

Just a few weeks ago when Jane Ann Jayroe came home to Laverne, she was just another college girl home for a visit with her parents and friends....Well, she is coming home to Laverne today. But it will be different, much different. This time she's coming home as the reigning Miss America and it's big doings in the old hometown...and rightly so.

Jane Ann today is climbing the arc of the rainbow...She's coming home to the plaudits of thousands of hometown and area friends. We wish for her every honor the day holds.

It was a carnival atmosphere in my hometown. Governor Henry Bellmon was on hand to welcome me. He had proclaimed Laverne the state capital for the day and officially proclaimed my parents as "Oklahoma Parents of the Year." My mother will never forgive herself for not inviting the governor into our home for a snack when he came to our front door just before the parade—that is what you do in Laverne for visitors. Many years later, I apologized to him, but Governor Bellmon is such a person of character that he said he never thought anything about it.

I was in the first car of an hour-long parade. Old timers said it was the first time Laverne ever had a parade with floats. One float watched by thousands of people who jammed the sides of the street carried my former basketball teammates. My grandparents rode in a specially decorated vehicle and my sister in another. The Future Homemakers of America float was a candle-studded birthday cake made of crepe paper. It was a few days early for my birthday.

I cried when I saw so many people along the parade route who had meant so much to me in my life. Painted signs in the windows along the street welcomed me in grand fashion. In the Ideal Grocery window was a sign that read, "Greets for the Ideal girl, Jane Jayroe." Wallenberg's sign said, "Congratulations to our 'fair lady.'" Ponda Rosa Floral's sign read, "A bokay for Jaynie." Even the post office had a sign, "Home address of Miss America, 73848."

After the parade, I held a press conference and attended a "Laverne only" reception for my family and friends from Laverne in the high school auditorium. We then walked to the football stadium where more than 6,000 people had gathered for a two-hour program that featured Governor Bellmon,

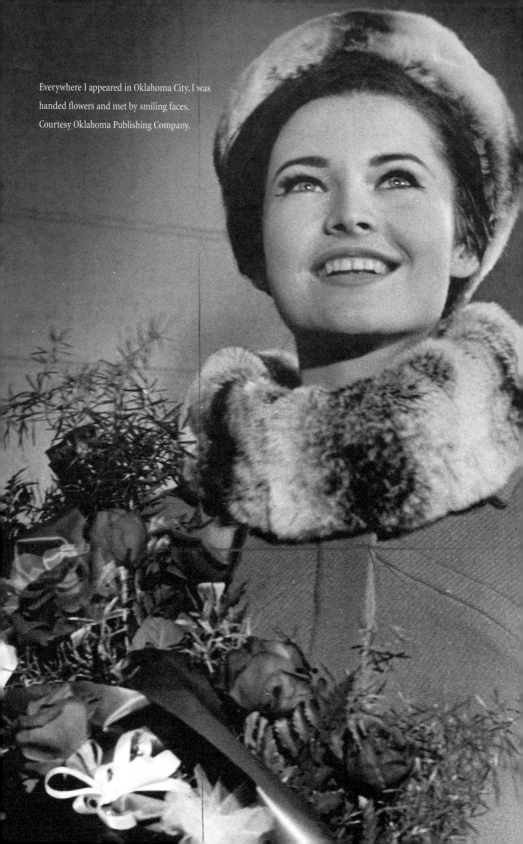

Everywhere I appeared in Oklahoma City, I was
handed flowers and met by smiling faces.
Courtesy Oklahoma Publishing Company.

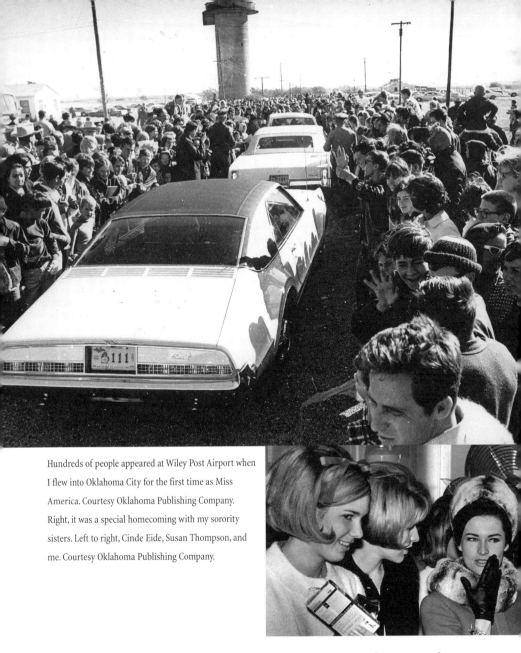

Hundreds of people appeared at Wiley Post Airport when I flew into Oklahoma City for the first time as Miss America. Courtesy Oklahoma Publishing Company. Right, it was a special homecoming with my sorority sisters. Left to right, Cinde Eide, Susan Thompson, and me. Courtesy Oklahoma Publishing Company.

Congressman Jed Johnson, Jr., Supreme Court Justice Robert Lavender, State Senator Leon Field, and State Representative Jack Harrison. On the platform were my parents, my Smith grandparents, Grandmother Jayroe, and my sister and her family.

After entertainment by a drill team from Clinton-Sherman Air Force Base and students from Oklahoma State University, I was introduced to the cheering throng of people. I told them that the homecoming they had given me was the greatest thrill next to winning the Miss America crown.

The next day I had a full schedule of performances in Oklahoma City. The capital city gave me a red carpet homecoming as I stepped from a jet at Wiley Post Airport just after noon. According to a newspaper story, there were more than 300 people at the airport. After still another meeting with reporters, I traveled to the OCU campus and met with students and faculty in the auditorium. On the way, I dedicated a new branch post office in Bethany and was blessed by the waves and cheers of hundreds of people.

Of course, being at OCU was heartwarming. This was my community of peers. One of the snap shot moments in my visual memory bank is when I walked on the stage at OCU to see people in the jam-packed auditorium yelling and clapping. In two years, I had been on that stage numerous times, but never alone. As I stood there with no back drop, no fellow contestants, no sorority sisters, I just received what they so generously gave. I hoped I would not have to speak, because I really was not very good at it.

I wanted to be articulate, profound, and able to communicate what they meant to me, but I usually just kind of blubbered and bungled something. I think I was sincerely grateful and noticeably touched by the outpouring of their enjoyment of our shared success. Those qualities seem to be enough at such gatherings to compensate for my lack of speaking skills.

After the appearance at the auditorium, my sorority sisters threw me a birthday party. It was nice to be around my friends.

That night, thousands turned out for a downtown Oklahoma City parade, my second parade in two days. Afterwards, I was honored at a huge banquet at the Skirvin Tower Hotel where pageant officials had arranged for me to stay with my parents. The Oklahoma City Chamber of Commerce presented me with a silver tea service that I still cherish today.

The three days in Oklahoma were among the greatest days of my life. It made me even prouder of my native state. I was determined to represent Oklahoma as well as I could for the remaining ten months of my fairy tale year as Miss America.

HENRY BELLMON

~ ~ ~ *"One of the finest days in my service as governor was to welcome Jane home to Laverne, on her first trip to Oklahoma after being crowned Miss America. The excitement of her neighbors who had seen her grow into a beautiful young lady was overwhelming."*

DR. MICHAEL ANDERSON

~ ~ ~ *"Jane is the quality of personhood that makes the place she lives come alive. Her God-given gifts of beauty and gracefulness are presented without fanfare or artificiality. I like the way she enjoys "walking the walk" not merely "talking the talk" of life. Benjamin Franklin said, "Never confuse motion with action." While many people just talk about doing things, Jane is a reflection of Franklin's idea—she has the ability to get important things done."*

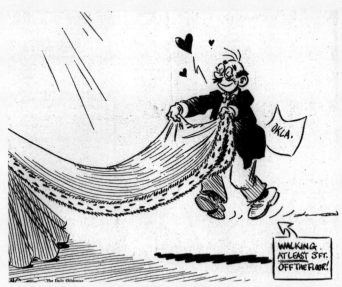

Newspaper cartoonists chronicled my time as Miss America.

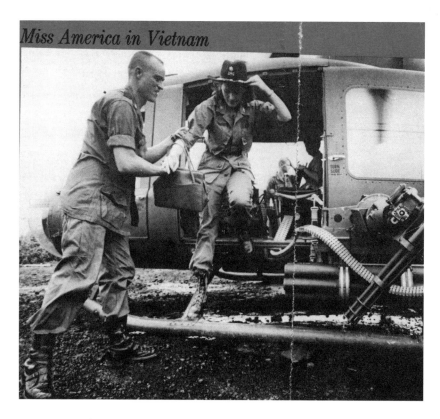

Miss America in Vietnam

In Vietnam, we rode in noisy, open-door helicopters. Everywhere we went, we received huge ovations. A military newspaper carried the photograph and a caption, "Jane Jayroe is not a military genius. And she wears a miniskirt, not a toga. But like the ancient Roman, Julius Caesar, she saw and she conquered. The divine Caesar merely demolished the bodies of the Gauls, whereas the diviner Miss Jayroe laid waste the hearts of her fellow Americans. Thousands of them paused in their search for a battlefield to enjoy the curves and talent of this Laverne, Oklahoma, brunette."

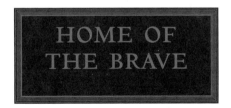

10

HOME OF THE BRAVE

*I*n traveling more than 200,000 miles as Miss America, mostly by air, I was destined to lose my luggage at least once. On one trip, trying to fly from Portland, Oregon, to Tulsa, I missed a fogged-in connecting flight in Denver, Colorado, and was rerouted all day. When I arrived in Tulsa, my luggage was nowhere to be found. Fortunately, I was in a city where I had friends and wore a borrowed gown, with no crown, at an appearance.

The next morning one piece of luggage turned up. It had actually arrived with me in Tulsa, but a young girl picked it up, thinking it was hers. Later, when I opened the suitcase, I found a note inside that she was sorry that I had been inconvenienced, but she was thrilled to have mistakenly carried Miss America's suitcase home with her.

In my year as Miss America, I was able to come home to Oklahoma several times. In November, 1966, I appeared at the 33rd annual convention of the Oklahoma Automobile Dealers Association where I was serenaded by some of my OCU classmates, the Surrey Singers.

My favorite Oldsmobile friends were in Oklahoma. Ed and Barbara Eskridge in Oklahoma City and Jackie and Barbara Cooper in Yukon were the best, both professionally and personally, among the many Oldsmobile dealers I appeared with across the country.

Many of my appearances as Miss America tested my resilience and resolve. Smiling and shaking thousands of hands really gets old. It was work, but I was paid well. However, there were other appearances at which I was overjoyed to make. In December, 1966, I spoke at the National 4-H Club

Congress in Chicago, Illinois. I was honored to appear and talk about my 4-H Club experience at Laverne.

I was scheduled to sing "Oklahoma!" for the audience. However, as I led the orchestra, I stopped the music and asked all the 4-H kids from Oklahoma to join me. I told the people, "You can't appreciate this song without hearing the words." All the Oklahoma delegates rose from their tables near the stage and helped me end the meeting with a rousing rendition of our state song.

In March, 1967, I came home again and appeared before a joint session of the Oklahoma legislature presided over by Lieutenant Governor George Nigh. My own legislators, Senator Leon Field and Representative Jack Harrison, had coauthored a legislative resolution commending me for being named Miss America.

I was again humbled by the response of my fellow Oklahomans. The gallery in the Oklahoma House of Representatives in the State Capitol was packed to the rafters. Governor Dewey Bartlett proclaimed the day "Jane Jayroe Day" in Oklahoma. I was presented a full set of Frankoma pottery. I never had a gift for speaking and there was never a second to prepare a word, so I have not a clue what I said at such a wonderful occasion—I am sure it was not profound. However, I am also sure that whatever I said was from the heart—and in Oklahoma, that seemed to be enough.

On a trip home to Laverne, I received a surprise gift. Bill Sizelove, a rancher who lived outside Laverne, gave me a quarter horse colt he had named "Miss America Miss." I had received at least 1,000 bouquets of roses in my first eight months as Miss America, but never a horse.

Another thrilling experience was the International Lions Club Convention in Chicago. I was part of the opening ceremonies. I walked into the packed convention hall carrying the American flag in full spotlight. It was a peak experience as I walked the full length of the arena while the National Anthem was playing.

I attended a lot of pageants and fashion shows in the United States, Canada, and Europe and rode in many parades. I threw out the first baseball to open the season for the Kansas City Athletics and conducted symphony orchestras. I lived in a hotel in New York City and loved the theater and shopping. I traveled daily, ate dishes of which I had never heard in the most sophisticated restaurants in the world, as well as fun down-home places such as Stone Crab Joe's. I gained weight with the joy of it all and really struggled to not outgrow my new clothing. Talking to people all the time really made me tired—eating was an escape and yummy diversion from the talking.

Whether it was a Snow Queen Festival in South Dakota at 19 degrees below zero, the Cherry Blossom Festival in Washington, D.C., with a visit from my friend and Speaker of the United States House of Representatives, Carl Albert, or a photo shoot in New York City with famous fashion photographer, Horst, life was an extended sprint with hardly a day off. My chaperones traded off every month, and they were each a gift to me in different ways.

My Christmas in Laverne was heavenly. I bought mother a mink stole. But nothing could have made us richer than just to be together with Judy and Don's little boy, Jace. People in Laverne were so considerate of my privacy. It was a welcome and holy holiday. The New Year began with a fun appearance at the Cotton Bowl in Dallas where I sat above the world on top of a huge Frito Lay float for the Cotton Bowl parade. Life was good.

I came to enjoy press conferences and appearances on televisions shows like the "Today Show" and "Match Game." On that game show, our team won handily even though some of my answers were considered funny because they were so Middle America. One example was completing the question, "On the way home from work, I stopped and picked up _____." I answered "a carton of milk" and the other celebrity guest answered "a six-pack of beer," which I guess was the more common answer on the east coast. Few people in western Oklahoma stopped for a six-pack on the way home from work. My family never did. My team on "Match Game" also put "milk," to the surprise of the host who had thought my answer was pretty funny.

In spite of all these glorious experiences, I missed home, especially my mother, and my girlfriends. Once in awhile, but not often, former contestants such as Miss North Carolina, or when I was in Oklahoma, Jeannie Alexander, Miss Pauls Valley, or Nancy Turk, Miss Ardmore, would be at an appearance. I craved their companionship, even if it was brief.

Being Miss America was a lonely existence. Even when I experienced a thrilling occasion there was no one to share it with personally or even by phone. Oklahoma was in a different time zone and my family and friends were already in bed by the time I arrived at my hotel.

By late spring, 1967, constant travel was getting to me. I was in Dillon, South Carolina, where I wrote in my diary, "I've lost all enthusiasm for these things. I'm not a person to these people—and when I get off a Piedmont puddle-jumper at 7:30 after starting at 11:00 that morning, I don't look like the person they expect to see. I'm ready to go home and go to work…to accomplish something…to do something besides smile! These people deserve more than me." I was just cranky, tired, and homesick.

One day in particular was horrible. I woke up sick, with 102-degree fever from a Black Plague vaccination for the Vietnam trip, and had to wait three hours in the Chicago airport where I went to the bathroom and cried. I flew to Little Rock, Arkansas, and made four appearances, then drove to nearby Hot Springs. In spite of being sick, they talked me into walking the runway for their pageant. I did not want to—but I did anyway. I was embarrassed to look so bad! Fortunately, I was able to participate fully by the final night. It was a great state pageant and they were very generous.

In April, Ban-Lon sent me to Europe for a two-week fashion tour with my dear friend and mentor, Lola Costigan Martin. This was Lola's final year as Ban-Lons' vice president of marketing and she was determined to show me Europe in a way to create lasting memories. She "did it up right," as we would say in Laverne.

In London, England, Dusseldorf, Germany, Paris, France, Zurich, Switzerland, Barcelona, Spain, and Rome, Italy, we did our work and played like crazy. Lola made sure I saw all the highlights for my education, but she made sure I experienced the culture, whether it was seeing the Pope at the Vatican, eating croissants at the top of the Spanish steps, dancing at the hottest clubs in London after attending the opera at Covent Garden, witnessing a bullfight in Spain, or strolling in Hyde Park in London. I loved almost everything—I really did not like the killing at the bullfight.

Traveling with us were Ban-Lon executives from Europe who added positively to every experience, especially a man named Farouk Moussa. We enjoyed huge press conferences in every city and my visit was often front page news.

In early July, I learned that my wish to visit American soldiers in Vietnam was coming true. Bob Hope had asked earlier in the year, and the pageant had declined. Miss America headquarters had worked out plans with the Department of Defense and the United Service Organizations (USO) for a 17-day visit in the war zone to entertain some 450,000 American troops. Scheduled to make the trip with me were Miss Alabama, Angeline Grooms; Miss Connecticut, Carole Ann Gelish; Miss South Carolina, Barbara Anne Harris; Miss Wisconsin, Sharon Mae Singstock, and Miss Maine, Ellen Warren.

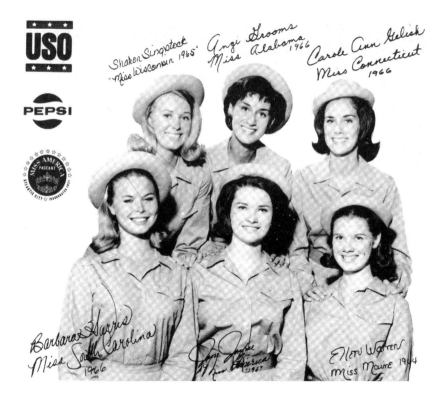

I had wonderful traveling companions on the USO tour to Vietnam. Front row, left to right, Miss South Carolina, Barbara Harris, me, and Miss Maine, Ellen Warren. In back, Miss Wisconsin, Sharon Singstock, Miss Alabama, Angi Grooms, and Miss Connecticut, Carole Ann Gelish.

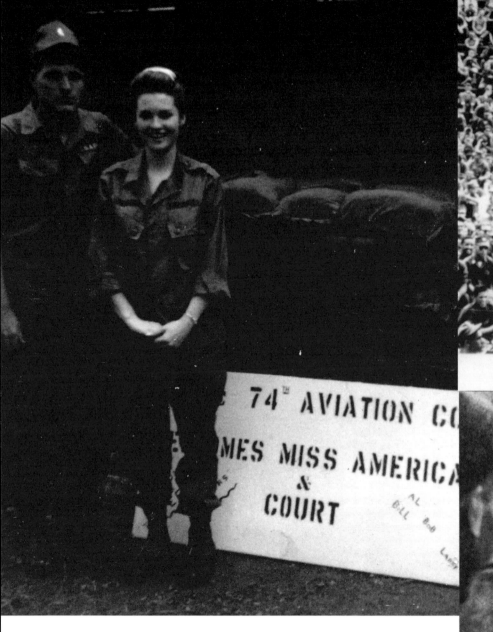

Above, it was really fun to see my cousin, Michael J. Smith, on the trip to Vietnam. Facing page, top, I was overwhelmed with joy and pride for America when I appeared before huge audiences of American heroes, our fighting men and women in Vietnam.

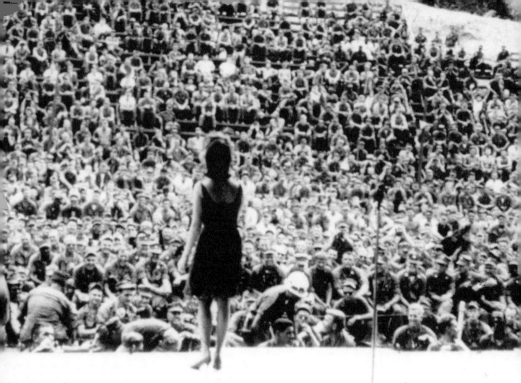

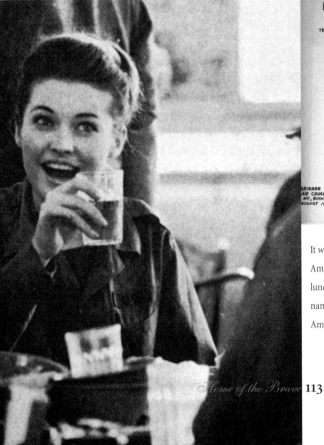

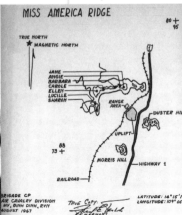

MISS AMERICA RIDGE

It was good to spend my time talking to American soldiers in Vietnam. Here I am having lunch with troops at Xuan Loc. The Army even named one of the hills around Binh Dinh "Miss America Ridge," in honor of our visit.

On August 14, actress Joan Crawford, representing our sponsor, Pepsi-Cola, and USO, took us to dinner at a very exclusive New York city restaurant and gave us lovely gifts. Mine was a bottle of Joy perfume. I was thrilled. She posed for photographs with us and launched us on our trip from New York City with 300 messages from parents and relatives of GIs in Vietnam. I was so excited as our airplane took off from John F. Kennedy Airport, headed for Travis Air Force Base in California where we would transfer to a military plane for the long trip to southeast Asia.

The press coverage of our trip to Vietnam was incredible. The war was getting a lot of negative press in America, and reporters seemed to welcome the change of pace of writing about beauty queens presenting our musical show, "What's Going On Back Home."

From California, we made an intermediate stop at Clark Air Force Base in the Philippines. My really good friend, Ellen Warren, Miss Maine, walked off the plane first and was mistaken for Miss America. The press followed her for a few minutes before they discovered their mistake. I loved every minute of it!

When we landed in South Vietnam's capital of Saigon, I entered a strange world of which I knew nothing—filth, barbed wire, sand bags, horrible smells, and fear everywhere. On the very first day we were there, we visited an Army hospital. The sight of young Americans with missing limbs and catastrophic injuries crushed my spirit.

We made at least two stops each day to entertain and just visit with soldiers. The Army assigned Captain Frank Lennon to escort our troupe around the country. Captain Lennon later told *Time* magazine:

> There I was, mushing around in the Central Highlands counting Viet Cong dead. I was the grubbiest man alive. Bad, really bad. After two days of no sleep, I went back to camp and sacked out on an air mattress in the mud. Then came a voice telling me to get up and go to Saigon to take care of Miss America. Not bad for a dream. Even better as the real McCoy. So I scraped off the mud and flew to Saigon to act as official escort for Jane Jayroe, the new Miss America.

In Vietnam, I have never been so close to death and violence, but never felt so protected and safe. We were traveling with America's finest, our classmates, our friends, our young men who had grown into soldiers overnight. I wrote my first letter to mother by flashlight under a mosquito net. Every 10 minutes or so, I heard bombs exploding in the distance.

The Army provided a guard at the door of our primitive housing, whether we stayed in a tent or barracks. We experienced all kinds of transportation on the ground and in the air. We flew in helicopters with no doors and machine guns on the side. The Chinook choppers were noisy, but we learned to sleep on them. It was a thrill to be catapulted off an aircraft carrier into the blue of the ocean and sky.

One of the highlights of my trip was seeing my cousin, Michael J. Smith of Turpin, who was assigned to the 34th Artillery Company at Bung Tau. The Army was aware he was my cousin and flew him to stay with me a few days. A television crew filmed a feature about Mike and me, so the family back home got to see him up close. Mike had been such a wonderful young man growing up—such a good student and great athlete. It hurt me inside to see him in the midst of all that killing and sadness. I cried when he had to be airlifted back to the front—I thought I might never see him again. Fortunately, he did survive and returned home to the Oklahoma Panhandle.

Whether we were in unknown Vietnamese villages with names like Cu Chi, Lai Khe, and Long Giao, or aboard the modern aircraft carrier, the USS *Constitution*, GIs showed up hours early to get as close as they could to the stage. Regardless of the weather, the men gathered by the thousands and gave us standing ovations for just walking on the stage. It was one of the most gratifying experiences of my life.

We had several funny experiences in the midst of challenging circumstances. Our producers in the United States thought it was cute to see American beauties dressed in military fatigues, so we did a couple of numbers in them. However, when our boys saw us dressed that way, they booed. That was the last thing they wanted to see. It did not take us long to change our performance—we wore our cute little dresses on stage regardless of how much they needed cleaning. A couple of our performances were in the rain, and the chiffon would shrink, making the dresses even shorter. It was not a problem for the cheering GIs.

Sometimes, in the midst of performing to cheering American boys, I would forget that the war was happening around us. However, there was always something to shock me back to reality. On the day we arrived on the aircraft carrier, three planes with their pilots and crews did not return from their mission.

On the long trip back to the United States, I spent a lot of time thinking about the war, the protests on American college campuses, and the thousands of healthy, young American boys who were risking their life and limb every day for me and all the millions who were living normal lives at home. I had seen the terror in which they lived, and have never been the same. I have never resented the protest of war because it is such a basic right we have as Americans. But I have little tolerance for how our soldiers were treated when they came home from Vietnam. They answered the call on their lives made by this country and that deserved respect and honor. To this day, I fight tears every time I see a news story about a Vietnam veteran.

The trip back home was full of emotion aboard the plane of military personnel that brought us home from Vietnam. We were exhausted—we were changed. When we saw the California coastline, we were overwhelmed with the beauty of America—it was so clean and free—and began singing "America." There was not a dry eye anywhere in sight.

For months after I returned, I received letters from GIs. Carl Belson, a member of the 173rd Airborne Brigade, wrote, "I was just sitting over here wondering what I was fighting for. Then you came to my mind, a beautiful symbol of our country. You are one of the reasons that we are over here, to keep people like you free!" The wonderful soldier ended his letter with the admonition, "Keep smiling—that alone will keep America beautiful!" I blushed when he told me that about 40 percent of the men in his brigade were from Oklahoma and they had adopted me for Christmas.

A Navy seaman aboard the USS *Intrepid* was so entranced with seeing Miss America and American girls, he had a photograph taken with me and sent me a copy. An officer aboard the Intrepid gave me wonderful compliments about my smiling. He wrote, "I have seen and spoken to you at least five times since you came aboard the ship and each time you spoke and smiled back. You seem to be just as happy to be here as the crew—there seems to be a smile upon each and every face since you have arrived." When I read the letter, I felt badly about ever not wanting to smile for anyone who wanted to meet Miss America.

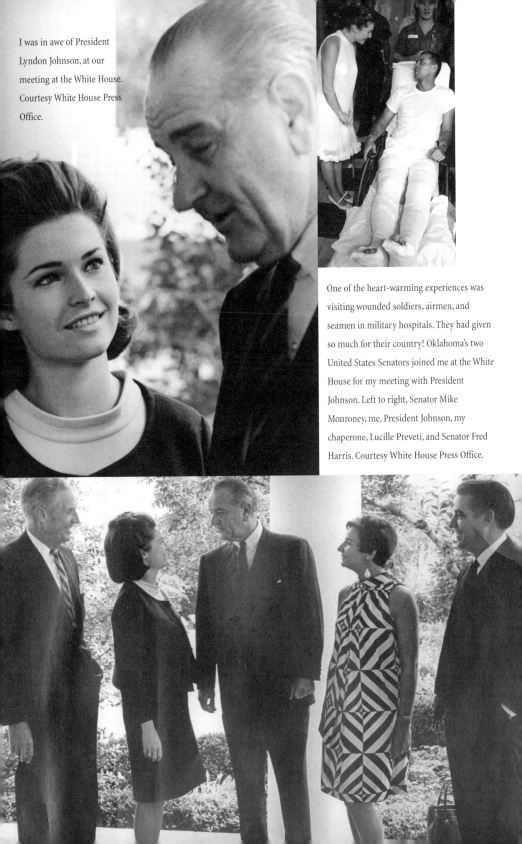

I was in awe of President Lyndon Johnson, at our meeting at the White House. Courtesy White House Press Office.

One of the heart-warming experiences was visiting wounded soldiers, airmen, and seamen in military hospitals. They had given so much for their country! Oklahoma's two United States Senators joined me at the White House for my meeting with President Johnson. Left to right, Senator Mike Monroney, me, President Johnson, my chaperone, Lucille Preveti, and Senator Fred Harris. Courtesy White House Press Office.

Other soldiers, airmen, and seamen wrote me such nice letters. Major Lewis Harrison said, "As days go by on the ship, it is hard at times to tell Sunday from Wednesday. But when you came aboard, the day could have been the Fourth of July, Christmas Day, or any special holiday!"

A few hours after we returned to New York City, we received a call from President Lyndon Johnson, inviting us to the White House. With almost no sleep in three days, my chaperone and I rallied for this summon to the White House

When I met with the president in the Oval Office at the White House, and he thanked me for going to Vietnam and asked me how our boys were doing, I was so awestruck I could not think of a single word to say. Fortunately, Oklahoma's two United States Senators soon joined us for the meeting so I did not have to say much except "fine!" I was completely unprepared for the deluge of reporters that descended upon me after I left the White House meeting. They wanted to know everything that was said. I remembered many of the eloquent words of appreciation of the president, but I could not remember anything important I had said to him. Casual conversations sure sound trivial when repeated!

I was ready for my year as Miss America to be over, although glamorous living, attention, and expense accounts were habit forming.

My focus changed in September, 1967, during pageant week in Atlantic City. Even though the new contestants showed me great respect, I really began taking a smaller role in the production. I took a final walk down the runway at Convention Hall in a beautiful gown, feeling so much more confident than I had a year before. When the new Miss America was crowned, I was simply a "former" Miss America. It was okay with me.

I reflected upon the year. Had I been exploited by the pageant system? Not at all. The Miss America institution had served me well, with amazing scholarships and travel to places I would never have seen. I met people who still inspire me. Sometimes I had felt like a generic doll that really was not quite pretty enough to be chosen. But I was extremely well paid for the work that I performed.

Sometimes I had acted like a rebellious teenager, hurrying off to chew gum behind closed doors. But other moments made the year so worthwhile—times of being hugged by a child with cerebral palsy who told me I made his world bright because I had a crown on my head. I had been treated like royalty in Europe, like the greatest American hero when I walked into a huge convention singing a patriotic song, and loved by literally hundreds of thousands of people during the previous 12 months.

I had received honor and respect I could never deserve. At the time, I only hoped that it would open doors and opportunities for me in the future and that I would someday learn how to make sense of it all.

I was finally free from the pre-determined daily schedules. As I prepared to return to OCU and resume my college class work, I wondered out loud, "What's at the end of the rainbow? I knew even though I could and would go home again—nothing would ever be the same. I asked myself, "Now, where does my life go?"

DON KERBY

~ ~ ~ *"Jane will always be remembered for visiting American troops in Vietnam during her reign. Seeing the Miss America ladies out on firebases and in the middle of combat was a wonderful reminder of what the United States is about. I will always cherish Jane's character and her Okie roots."*

TOM E. LOVE

~ ~ ~ *"By definition Miss America is possessed of great physical beauty. Add to that overwhelming fame and it would seem you have a situation that would lead to being quite full of one's self. Beautiful and famous Jane is—full of herself she is not. I did not know Jane before she became Miss America but I would bet she is the same person who grew up in Laverne. She is one of Oklahoma's state treasures."*

ED AND BARBARA ESKRIDGE

~ ~ ~ *"We first met Jane when she came to a reception for her at our Oldsmobile showroom. Oldsmobile was the pageant sponsor. She was a huge draw—everyone from Oklahoma was ready to cheer her on and eager to see her in person. She won everyone's heart and we were so proud of her."*

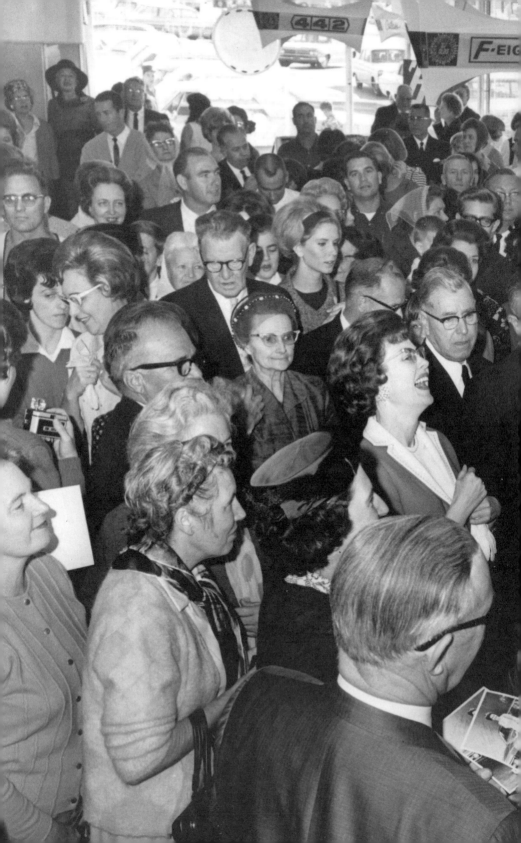

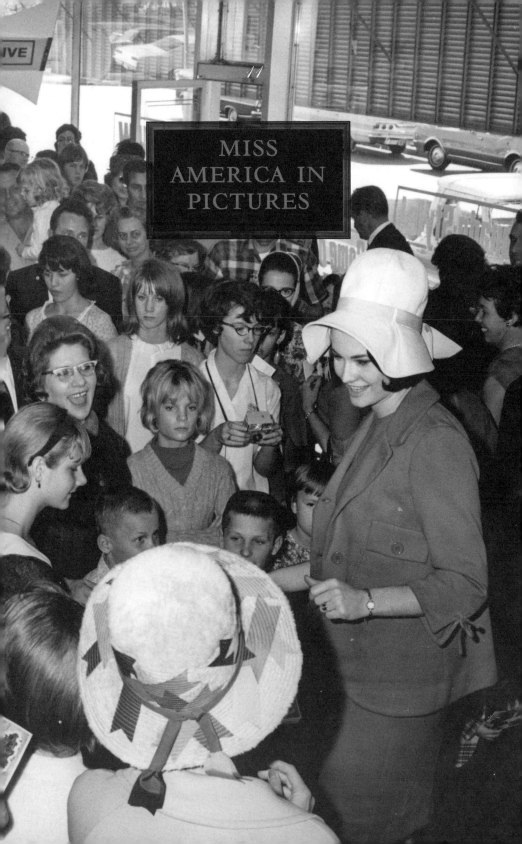

MISS AMERICA IN PICTURES

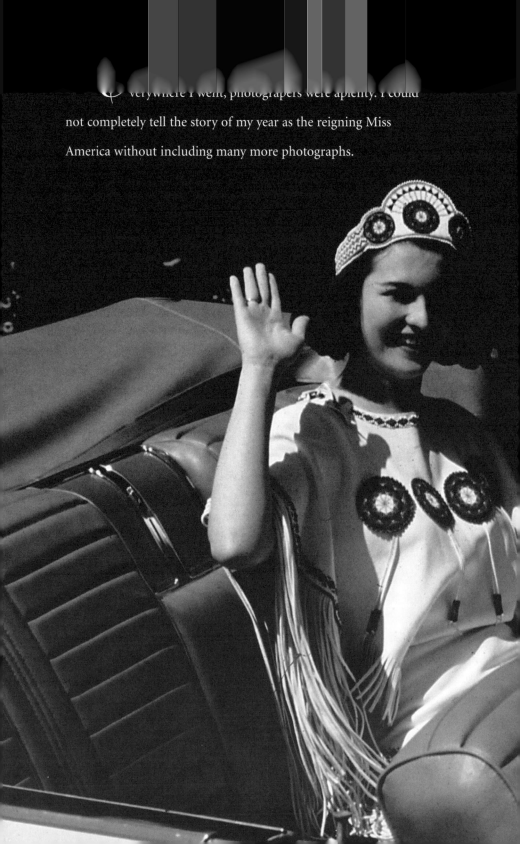

$\mathscr{E}$verywhere I went, photographers were aplenty. I could not completely tell the story of my year as the reigning Miss America without including many more photographs.

I rode in a parade in Muskogee, Oklahoma, dressed in a Native American dress they gave me. My home state honored me by posting "Home of Miss America" signs at each highway entrance to the state. Probably the only "Home of Miss America" sign that still exists is located on the ranch of Granville Chandler near Broken Bow. After visitors questioned whether Miss America actually lived on the ranch, Chandler named one of his pet pigs "Miss America," so the sign would be correct. My mother kept a map of my Miss America travels in her fifth grade classroom at Laverne. Preceding pages: I was surrounded by well wishers at the Eskridge Oldsmobile showroom on South Walker Avenue in Oklahoma City in 1967.

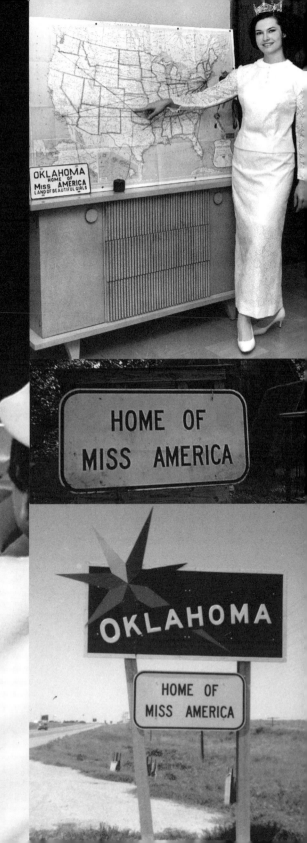

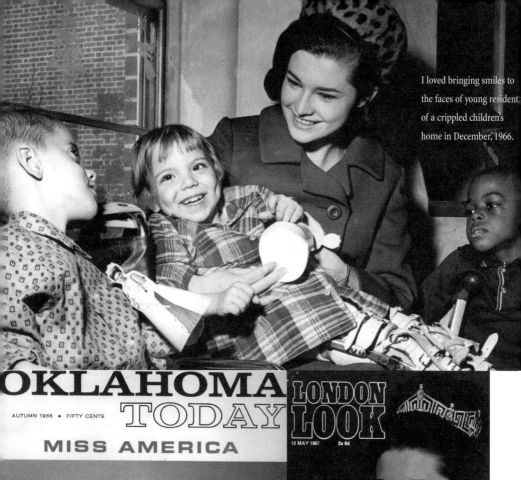

I loved bringing smiles to the faces of young residents of a crippled children's home in December, 1966.

AUTUMN 1966 • FIFTY CENTS

OKLAHOMA TODAY

MISS AMERICA

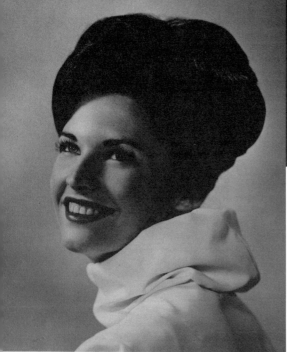

LONDON LOOK

13 MAY 1967   2s 6d

WHAT MISS AMERICA IS WEARING TO VISIT LONDON

WHAT'S ON ALL OVER TOWN AND EVERYWHERE TO GO

Left, soon after I was crowned Miss America, *Oklahoma Today* magazine featured me on its cover. Courtesy Oklahoma Department of Tourism and Recreation. Above, I made the cover of a magazine in London during the European tour of spring 1967.

MISS JAYNE JAYROE

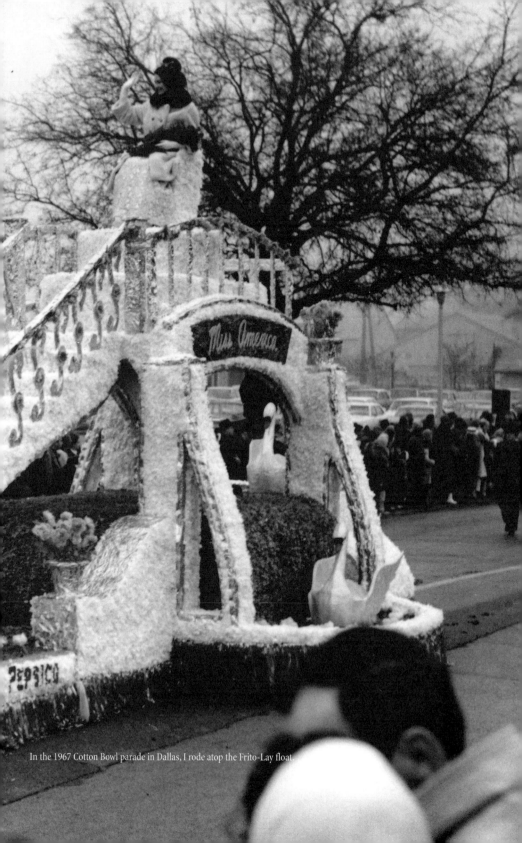

In the 1967 Cotton Bowl parade in Dallas, I rode atop the Frito-Lay float.

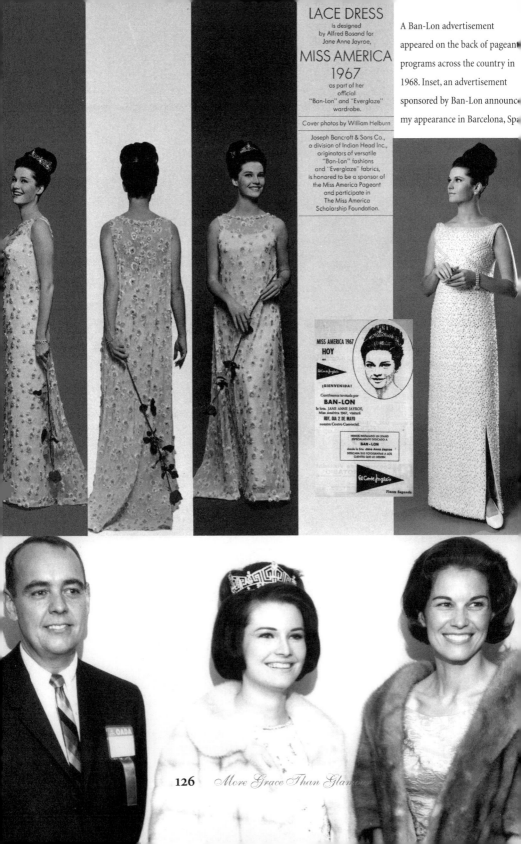

A Ban-Lon advertisement appeared on the back of pageant programs across the country in 1968. Inset, an advertisement sponsored by Ban-Lon announced my appearance in Barcelona, Spain.

More Grace Than Glamour

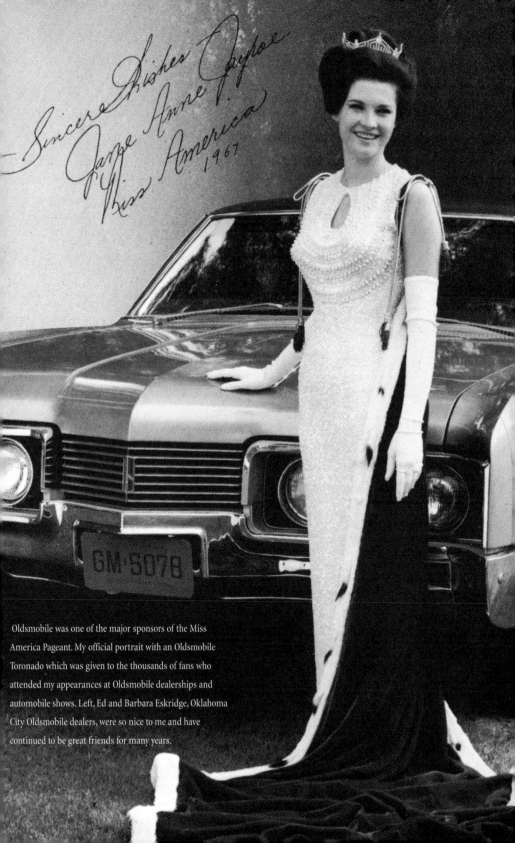

Sincere Wishes Jane Anne Jayroe Miss America 1967

Oldsmobile was one of the major sponsors of the Miss America Pageant. My official portrait with an Oldsmobile Toronado which was given to the thousands of fans who attended my appearances at Oldsmobile dealerships and automobile shows. Left, Ed and Barbara Eskridge, Oklahoma City Oldsmobile dealers, were so nice to me and have continued to be great friends for many years.

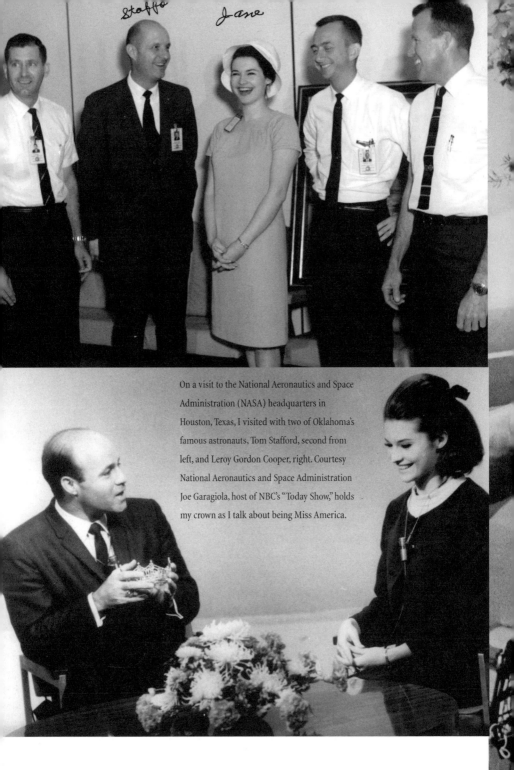

Stafford   Jane

On a visit to the National Aeronautics and Space Administration (NASA) headquarters in Houston, Texas, I visited with two of Oklahoma's famous astronauts, Tom Stafford, second from left, and Leroy Gordon Cooper, right. Courtesy National Aeronautics and Space Administration Joe Garagiola, host of NBC's "Today Show," holds my crown as I talk about being Miss America.

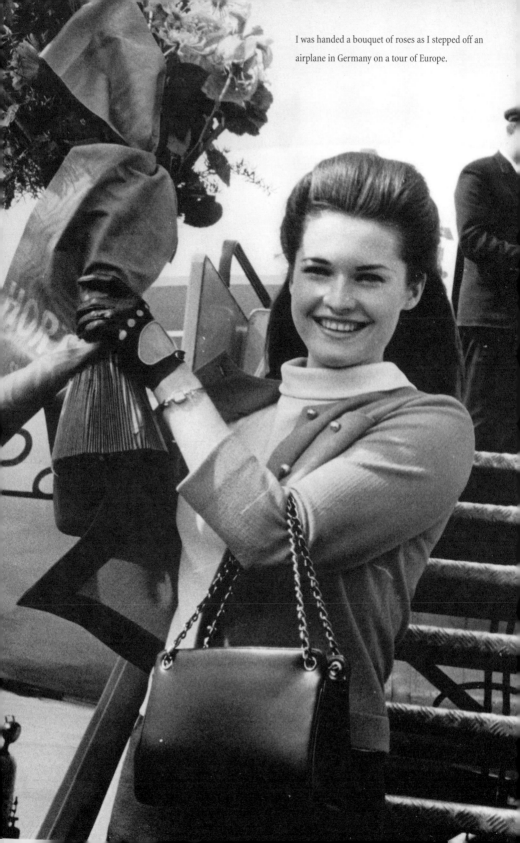

I was handed a bouquet of roses as I stepped off an airplane in Germany on a tour of Europe.

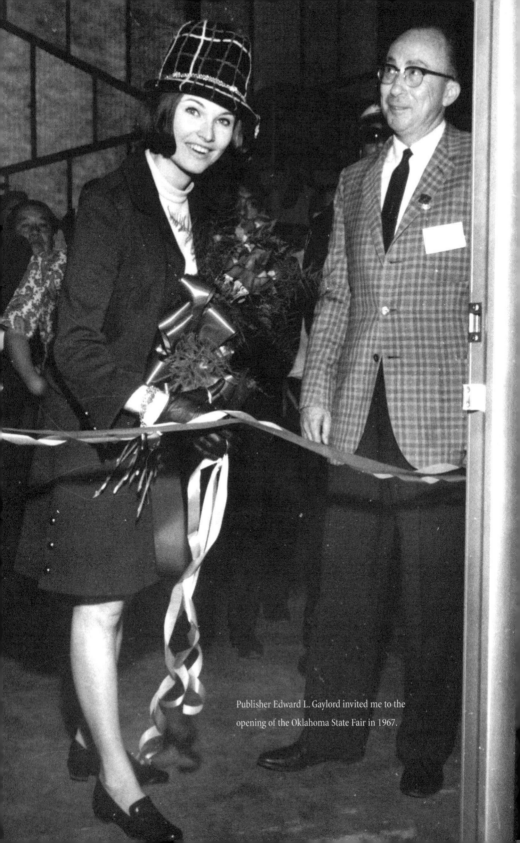

Publisher Edward L. Gaylord invited me to the
opening of the Oklahoma State Fair in 1967.

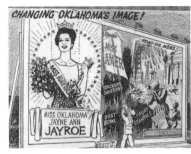

Below, Mr. and Mrs. Dick Pope, owners of Cypress Gardens in Florida were great supporters of the Miss America Pageant and invited Miss America to their beautiful location each year. Left, a newspaper cartoonist honored me by suggesting that I was changing Oklahoma's image.

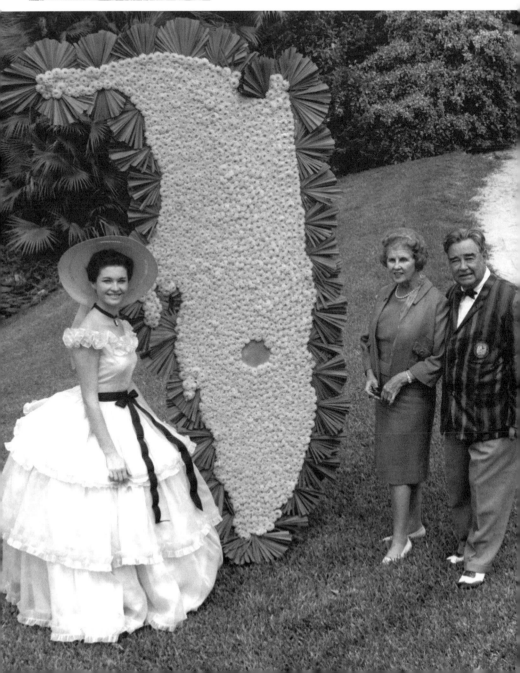

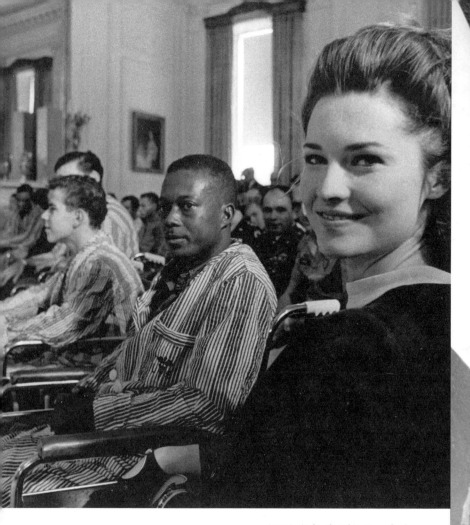

I was invited to the White House for the
signing of legislation that increased
benefits for veterans and made it easier for
wounded veterans to receive the best in
medical care. Courtesy White House Press
Office. Right, at the end of my year as Miss
America, I congratulated the new Miss
America, Debra Barnes, Miss Kansas.

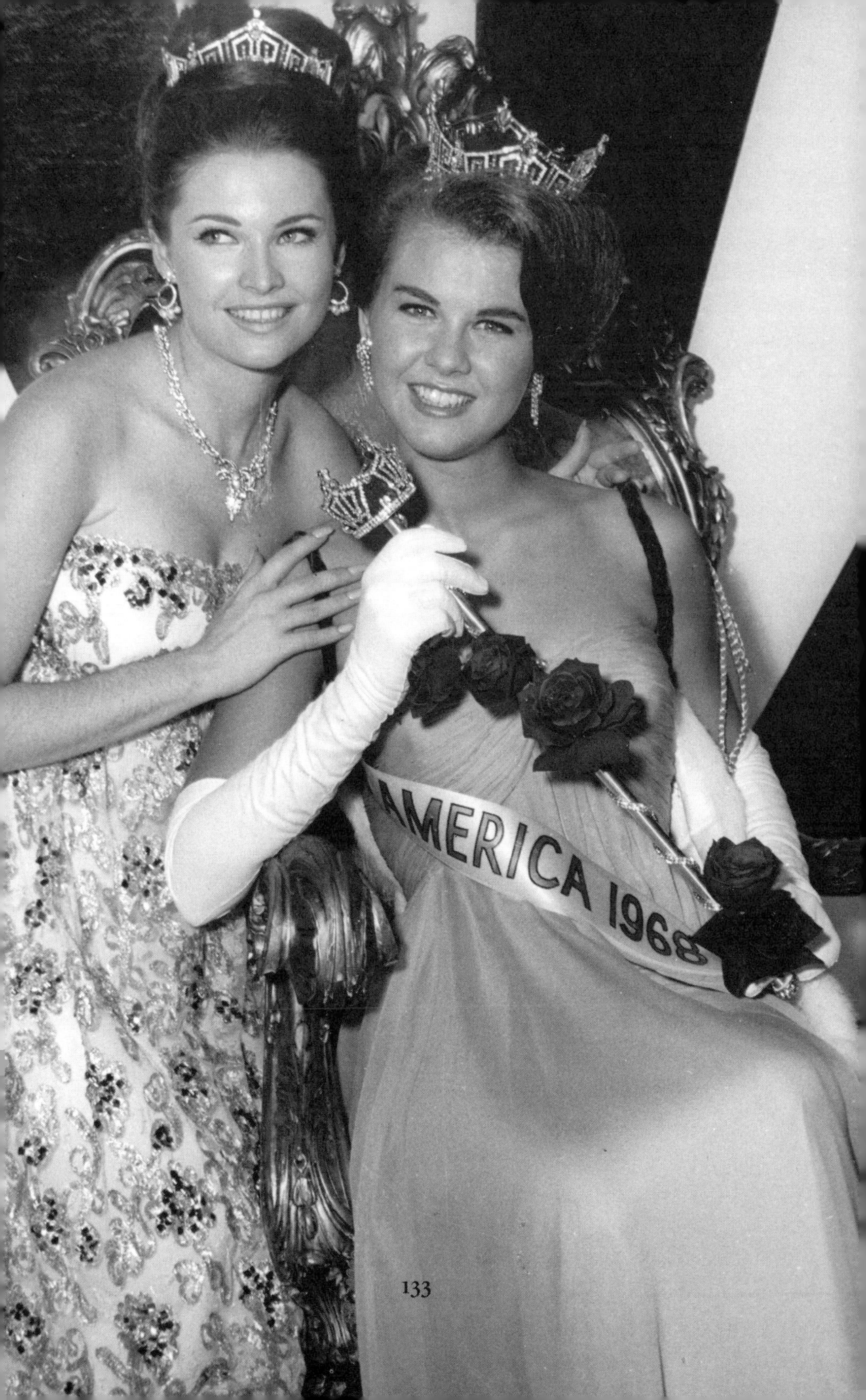
AMERICA 1968

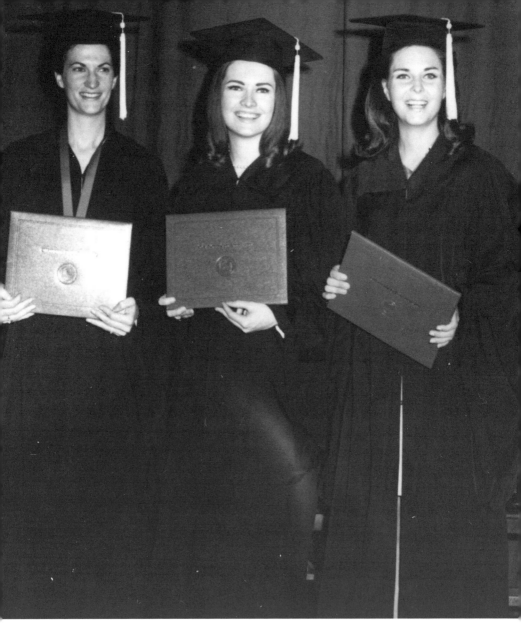

I graduated in 1969 from Oklahoma City University with a bachelor's degree in music education. Left to right, Sue Wells, me, and Beverly Drew.

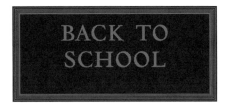

12

BACK TO SCHOOL

*M*y new life had begun the Sunday morning after the Miss America Pageant when I passed the crown on to Debra Barnes, Miss Kansas. It felt as if a giant load had been lifted from my shoulders. As wonderful as the year had been, now I was totally free to laugh and giggle and be myself with my family.

The only negative part of my first days as a "former Miss America" was the result of a reporter getting chummy with my father during the week of the pageant in Atlantic City. There was never a formal interview, but my dad felt comfortable with the reporter and innocently mentioned many of the frustrations I had shared only with my parents about the loneliness and demand of the Miss America schedule. Daddy never saw the reporter writing anything down, so he kept telling him everything, including, "When the pageant's over, they will drop Janie like a hot potato!"

No one thought anything about the conversations until Dad's comments showed up in a front page story. It appeared I was bitter at the Miss America Pageant officials and that I had been wronged by them. To make matters worse, the part about the supposed conflict was picked up by United Press International (UPI) and distributed worldwide. From the UPI story, readers got the impression that a terrible tempest had raged between the pageant and me—which was totally untrue.

I unsuccessfully tried to make amends with the pageant office. Our relations had been strained from the time of the dinner the evening following my crowning as Miss America, and this new wave of publicity was about as welcome as the measles.

I ran from reporters back in Oklahoma. The press had been wonderful to me during my reign, but I did not want to respond to this story. I wanted to run home--I just needed hugs from good friends at OCU, a quick fix at the Split-T, my favorite hamburger place in Oklahoma City, and a trip to see family and friends in Laverne.

I did not understand why Mother kept hurrying me along on the trip to Laverne. We had started the trip late, and even though it was midnight, I did not care—I was no longer on the pageant's printed schedule.

When we hit the six-mile-corner outside Laverne, I was shocked and delighted to see hundreds of people waiting to welcome me home. No wonder my mother had hurried me! The people had stood for hours by the highway, just to let me know in their own personal and private way how proud they were of "their Janie." With no television cameras or reporters in sight, it was a wonderful moment to share my life with my community.

I was home just long enough to trade evening gowns for blue jeans, glance at the stacks of souvenirs from my world travels, and pack my new stereo with towels, sheets, and causal clothing. Beautiful suits, hats, and gloves were no longer the daily uniform.

Without the fanfare that had driven my life for the past year, I moved back into the dormitory at OCU a few days later, just in time for fall semester classes. I was so glad to be back around people my own age. I had so missed just being a 19-year-old college student. During a brief interview with a reporter, I said, "I want to be an individual—not a title. I think people will begin to accept me as just me."

My wish for anonymity did not come true. On the first morning of class, I went to the student union for breakfast. I heard people whispering everywhere. All I could pick out of the whispers were "Jane" and "Miss America." I was totally embarrassed. I had always been shy and the past year had not changed that.

I thought I surely would drop my tray or fall over my feet if the whispers continued. Attention was nice when I was performing, but not at 7:00 a.m. in the cafeteria when I was half asleep and without makeup.

Even though I had already bought a meal ticket, and loved breakfast, I never ate in the cafeteria again. I wanted to turn out the stage lights, to do my own thing, and to get married, although there was no one on the scene for my immediate future. I did not know what else to do.

A few days after I began classes, I was asked to speak to about 800 coeds at Central State College in Edmond. I talked a lot about my trip to Vietnam and urged the girls to write to American servicemen. On the way back to my dorm, I began thinking about how my life had changed. I knew it would never be the same again.

I still thought about the dumb question, "How does it feel to be Miss America?" that had been asked me at nearly every stop along the way. There had been no chemistry change, no alteration of my genes, no royal transfusion, and basically no training. I was always Jane Anne Jayroe. Life had been incredibly altered by the contest I had entered.

I had assumed that dating would be easy once I returned to OCU. Although I wanted to be dated for being the person I had been, rather than for being Miss America, dating was difficult and uncomfortable. Many boys were afraid of asking me out. Even if they had asked, I would have been self conscious about going.

Rick Schuerman, the guy I had been dating when I went to Atlantic City, had received a lot of publicity as my "boyfriend." Unfortunately, the publicity had embarrassed our relationship beyond repair.

Even without an active dating life, I was having a ball. My financial package from my year as Miss America had made me rich in my eyes. No longer was paying tuition and room and board a chore for the family. I had the extra money to be able eat at the finest restaurants in Oklahoma City. The financial freedom gave me a sense of peace, not worrying about the future.

I also believed that surely Prince Charming would show up and take over my life. I really just wanted a simple life, and someone to love. I sometimes wished that I could be the type of person like Mary Ann Mobley, Miss America 1959, who took her scholarship money and headed back to college, totally with a career in mind. That was not me. For the moment, I could not concentrate on a career. I just wanted to catch up on fun and being young.

And I did—it was a great year of my life. I had so much of the attention of being Miss America, plus the people and places I treasured. I had great friends, classes, professors, and a new car. I felt like F. Scott Fitzgerald's Zelda, wild and high on the excitement of the moment.

I continued with my major in music education, even though I knew I would never teach. After much urging from Lee Allan Smith, I joined the staff of WKY Radio and Television in Oklahoma City as community relations coordinator, a newly-created position. I was supposed to visit communities to determine how WKY could better serve its listeners and viewers.

My first assignment was conducting an interview with Governor Dewey Bartlett and First Lady Ann Bartlett from the governor's mansion. I did not make as much out of the WKY opportunity as I could, because the only thing on my mind was falling in love, getting married, and living a charmed life like my parents had.

I was looking for someone who was more ambitious and more determined than I. If I could have written a classified ad for a husband, it would have read:

Former Miss America wants modern day hero. Must be strong, self-directed, dynamic, and full of energy. Also handsome, Protestant, and a Democrat. Rewards include submissive wife with stars in her eyes, humble, but successful background, sick of dressing up and wearing makeup. Loves novels, old movies, sloppy house shoes, and sleeping late.

In the end, I considered only one applicant, Paul Henry Petersen. His credentials were wonderful. He had been student body president at the University of Oklahoma, president of his fraternity, and intended to enroll in the OU School of Law as soon as he completed his business degree. He had graduated from U.S. Grant High School in Oklahoma City.

Our mutual friend, Cinde Eide, had put us together, hoping that a relationship between Paul and me would revitalize her former relationship with Paul's best friend, Craig Hoster. That part of the plan fizzled, but Paul and I became quite an item even before our first date.

Paul sent roses and a cute card saying I had won a phone call from him. I became his biggest project. Every date was well planned, including first class flights to Dallas for entertainment. I was swept off my feet, ecstatic, floating on clouds of romantic illusion.

On Valentine's Day, Paul asked me to marry him. Even though we had just been dating for a few months, I quickly said yes. The engagement remained a secret only for a couple of weeks. Everyone was talking about it, so I decided to make a public announcement on February 26. I told reporters, "It was such a good secret but I am surprised it lasted this long."

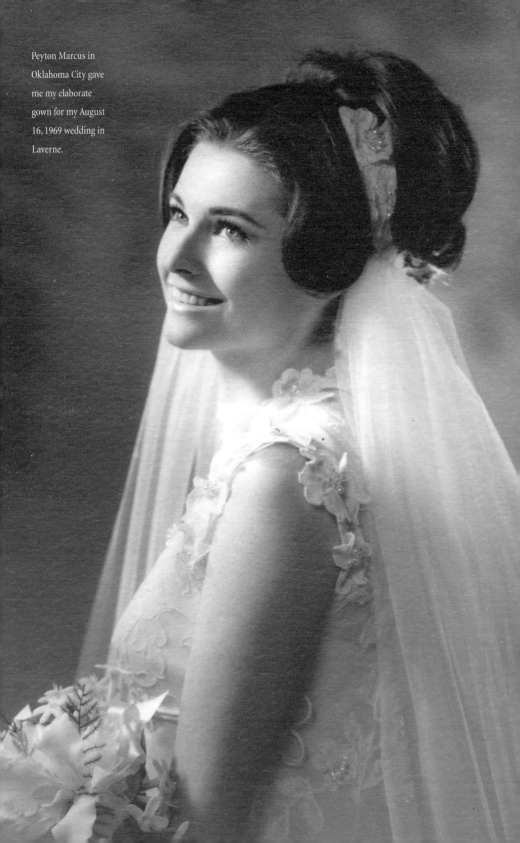

Peyton Marcus in
Oklahoma City gave
me my elaborate
gown for my August
16, 1969 wedding in
Laverne.

We decided upon August 16, 1969, as the date for the wedding. I just about worked my mother and sister to death to plan the wedding at my home church, First Methodist Church, in Laverne. Paul had graduated from OU in May and I was planning to enroll at OU to study radio and television in the fall, even though I also wanted to continue to study voice at OCU and complete my music education degree.

The wedding was like a fairy tale. My parents made everything perfect. I felt like a beautiful princess in my hometown. It was a great starring role without any competition. My former pastor, Reverend Leonard Gillingham, came from Albuquerque, New Mexico, from his present church assignment.

After the wedding, Paul and I spent a delightful honeymoon in Colorado. We then returned to a cute duplex in Norman for him to begin law school and me to continue my education and just be a wife, and hopefully, a mother. I had always wanted to be married—and now I was. Surely such a charmed beginning would continue with happily ever after.

DAVID L. BOREN

~ ~ ~ *"Jane is one of the most articulate and effective good will ambassadors the state has ever had. She is a person of strong character and great depth who knows Oklahoma's history and truly shares its bedrock values. The most important thing about Jane to me is that she is the same caring, generous, and sincere person "off camera" or "off stage" in her personal times as she is in front of an audience. Her public image as "the girl next door" who truly cares about others is a completely accurate reflection of the real person."*

LIEUTENANT GOVERNOR MARY FALLIN

~ ~ ~ *"Jane has been one of our state's most visible citizens for four decades now, from the most high-profile role one can imagine to a lot of behind the scenes work on behalf of community organizations and worthy causes. She is one of those people you think of first when you consider a list of Oklahomans who have made a profound difference for good."*

DICK AND SALLY BURPEE

~ ~ ~ *"Jane is a wonderful and talented ambassador for Oklahoma. She truly loves the state and its people. Jane has a "glow" to her countenance that causes others to gravitate to her. In spite of her public persona, she is unassuming, very approachable, and possesses that rate ability to make others feel important and good about themselves."*

JIM CLARK

~ ~ ~ *"One you get to know Jane a little, you quickly discover that her outward beauty is easily eclipsed by her inner beauty. Her most remarkable traits come from the inside. She uses all these traits to represent Oklahoma in such a grand and selfless way. She could have left Oklahoma—but she did not. She could have chosen to rest on her past accomplishments—but she did not. She could have retired from the public arena—but she did not. She could have said "no" many times—but she did not. And because she did not, Oklahoma is a better place, and those of us who have been blessed to cross her path are in a better place too."*

BOB FUNK

~ ~ ~ *"Jane is an Oklahoma treasure. From the time that she served as mistress of ceremonies at a surprise "This is your life" dinner sponsored by my employees, I have been a great admirer of this engaging woman of grace and panache. We are fortunate that she came back home to contribute so much to our state."*

JUDGE ROBERT HENRY

~ ~ ~ *"I first met Jane at a sing-a-long at my home. I had remembered her fabulous conducting skills made famous in the Miss America pageant. I had forgotten what a talented singer she was.*

Jane is a wonderful person. Her beauty is certainly not skin deep. She is naturally kind and compassionate, probably from her family and western Oklahoma roots. Grace is a good word to describe this inner talent.

Jane's major contribution to Oklahoma has been to remind this state of the basic decency of its people and to challenge them to go for the gold. She has excelled in every endeavor she has entertained. Her proficiency belies the arduous effort behind the success. She makes it look easy, but it is not and was not. Her model shows Oklahomans that talent and very hard work will take you a long way. And, she is a great person to have at a sing-a-long."

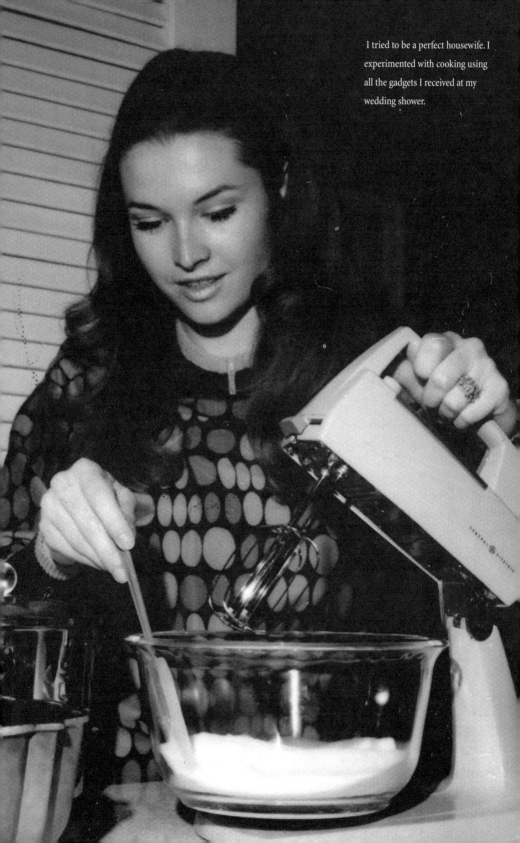

I tried to be a perfect housewife. I experimented with cooking using all the gadgets I received at my wedding shower.

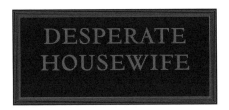

13

from the first day of marriage, I depended totally on Paul. Looking back, it was not good for the marriage, but I depended upon him to talk for us, to make all financial decisions, and literally plan our life. I was truly a completely submissive wife to a husband I had known less than a year. It never crossed my mind that my lack of participation in family decisions would have dire consequences. All I knew was that I was riding off on a white horse in the arms of my husband to Camelot where beauty queens and handsome men lived happily ever after.

My eyes may have been shielded, but my heart was hooked to a dream. I believed there was no need for me to speak for myself, nor have input into our plans. There was no need for planning or to be involved in anything except my marriage. I assumed that because marriage had been my ultimate goal, everything else would just happen. My parents had taken care of me, the Miss America managers had taken care of me, and now it was my husband's turn. I would be loving, kind, and faithful.

Paul began law school at OU and we lived comfortably in our duplex in Norman. I thought I was doing everything right to be a perfect wife. I kept a full pantry just like my mother and cooked us into chubbiness. For months after the wedding, I experimented with each piece of household equipment I received at the wedding shower. I even did the laundry every other day at a nearby laundromat.

Even though I did not perform some of the household chores very well—like ironing and cleaning—I was playing house, and it was great—for the moment. The first year of marriage flew by. I drove from Norman to Oklahoma City five days a week and graduated from OCU with a degree in music education, with a teaching certificate—neither of which I would ever use.

Our agenda was Paul's agenda. He either studied day and night or worried day and night about studying. Although neither of us realized it at the time, both of us felt that being married to me meant a lot to live up to.

However, at the time, my intensity was directed at being the best wife anyone could ever have. I sparingly agreed to personal appearances as a former Miss America. The extra money was great and the appearances were good for my ego. It also meant we could buy a washer and dryer. Paul did not want me to work outside the home, and I did not need to because I had saved $50,000 from my earnings as Miss America. It was certainly enough to support us through law school. The result was that he focused totally on his education—and I had nothing to do.

So I piddled, and enrolled in a few classes toward a master's degree. I watched a lot of day time television. But piddling takes it toll. I did not seem to fit in anywhere—not in the university community, among law wives, and certainly not in my major education field of teaching. I had completed a semester of student teaching in my last year at OCU and knew that teaching was not my cup of tea. As a child, I had loved the stories of my grandmother teaching in a one room schoolhouse on the prairie. And, my mother and father were lifetime teachers. My sister was an outstanding teacher. But teaching was not for Janie.

I spent every Friday in a funk because our weekends had become so depressing. Marriage was nothing like my dreams. Surely it would get better after three years of law school and Paul beginning practice. Surely there would be a new house to plan and furnish, an occasional night out, a morning at church, and a baby to love.

I would have an occasional respite that was fun, like a musical program I participated in at OU. I met Cleta Deatherage, a feisty blonde who loved to laugh. Cleta was later a strong voice in Oklahoma politics and served in the Oklahoma House of Representatives. Allen Hollingsworth was the drummer of the group. He became one of the outstanding breast cancer specialists in Oklahoma, as well as a successful author. Mark Houston was

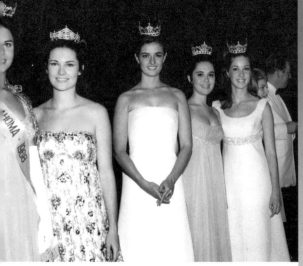

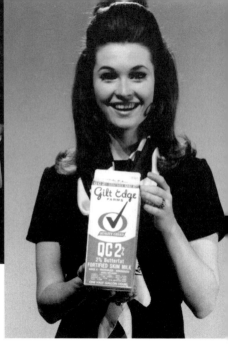

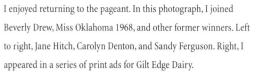

I enjoyed returning to the pageant. In this photograph, I joined Beverly Drew, Miss Oklahoma 1968, and other former winners. Left to right, Jane Hitch, Carolyn Denton, and Sandy Ferguson. Right, I appeared in a series of print ads for Gilt Edge Dairy.

the pianist and co-directed the group with Cleta. Mark became my accompanist for the next ten years. He died much too soon. I loved Mark—he was so creative and such a dear person.

Finally, my lack of regular activity forced me to try musical theater. Even though it had been my first love for as long as I could remember, the thought of auditioning made me anxious. No matter how many stages I had been on, auditioning for a part was different. It was still necessary to walk on stage with hundreds of others and perform. I had always thought of auditions as a parade of one vulnerable body after another—no applause, no kind words. How I hated auditions!

I talked myself into auditioning for a part in "The Boyfriend," a Jewel Box Theater presentation in Oklahoma City. Carveth Osterhaus was directing the play. Carveth and his wife, Kay Creed, were both OCU graduates and were my musical theater idols.

It was hard for me to audition with people who two years before had lined up to see me as Miss America. I knew I could sing, but was I good enough to be cast in a role with no prior experience in theater? Even though I was self-conscious, I desperately needed musical theater to survive.

I overcame my pride and took a tiny chorus role in the Lyric production.

I loved the show, although my miniscule part was tough on my ego. The cast was talented and totally fun to work with. Curt and Claire Schwartz, Debbie Giannopoulos, Susan and Don Detrick, Barbara Berard, Jane Hall, Mary Gordon Taft, Steve Coker, Cyde Martin, and David Anderson all made me feel welcome.

Actually, my pride was not my number one problem—fear was. Even though I had flown more than 250,000 miles in my year as Miss America, I was afraid to drive 30 miles from Norman to Oklahoma City for rehearsals and performances at night. I kept remembering traveling with a chaperone and my several scares from people obsessed with Miss America. Mobs had rocked my car, and periodically some unstable character would send a scary letter or, even worse, make a scary phone call. Driving alone at night was something I had never done—and it petrified me. And, there were no cell phones. But, if I was to be involved in musical theater, I had to drive. Paul could not help me because he was studying, either at home or in the library. So, I carefully locked my car doors and prayed the car would not break down on the highway between the theater and home.

I sang, danced in the chorus, and worked hard. I never complained, was always on time, and did my best to be the best. I needed to prove to myself and to those who were watching that I could do more. I wanted them to know that I could be in plays like *Oklahoma!* or *The Sound of Music,* even though it might mean more auditioning.

Soon, hard work paid off—I landed the role of Maria in *The Sound of Music,* produced by Lyric Theater in Oklahoma City with Bill Davidson as Captain Von Trapp, Mary Hudson as Mother Abbess, and a gaggle of delightful children. Lyle Dye was the director.

It was such fun—I loved every minute of it. For the first time since high school, I was performing in front of people I knew—peers, friends, family, faculty—Oklahomans.

For three years, musical theater was a wonderful distraction from my deep empty feelings. It was a haven, a cloud where I could park and play. It was a combination of friends, performing and belonging. It was like playing on the basketball team in the state finals again. It was being a cheerleader or part of the singing group I missed.

When Paul completed law school and passed the bar examination, he joined a prestigious law firm. We took off to make our nest in Tulsa, where life would surely get on track with a home, an improved marriage, and a baby that I so desperately wanted. Instead, my shyness almost delivered a knock-out punch.

I had never gotten over my shyness from childhood. Even though I could produce a Miss America smile and seem to be totally calm and in control on the outside, my stomach was doing flip flops. Making small talk was an art I had not learned well, and I was totally unable to wing anything. About the only way I could cover up my shyness was to let others initiate the contact. I would have died if I had been forced to approach a person cold and introduce myself.

Performing was different. I had butterflies, but they went away once I was on stage. I may have been so tired that I could hardly climb the stairs to where I was performing, but once the curtain opened, and the lights went on, I was front and center.

One of the great joys of playing Maria in "The Sound of Music" at the Lyric Theater in Oklahoma City was the interaction with all the delightful children.

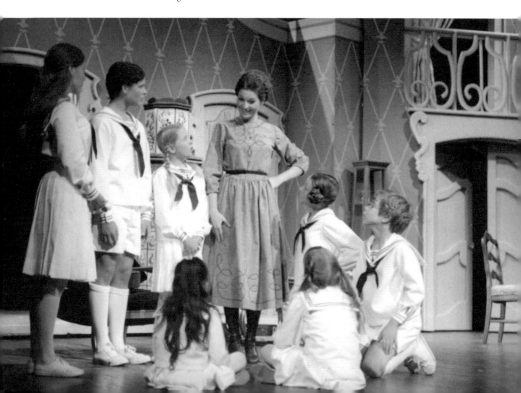

None of my previous experiences in my life was any help when I moved into a new town in the role of wife of an ambitious junior lawyer. No one took the initiative to meet me or include me. They probably thought I wanted to be left alone, especially when I never gave any indication of wanting to know people, have parties, or volunteer for any community activity.

The isolation was devastating. I grew stale and continued to pull the walls around me tighter and tighter until the smallest of steps outside required unusual courage. I saw how other people seemed to be so active, involved, and happy. I could never tell any of them that I was hurt and lonely—that knowledge would let them see my lack of purpose in life. I was so disappointed in myself—I had always been something—and now I was nothing. After having been given such a great gift of Miss America, how could I provide an encore that would not disappoint people?

I still received calls to be the master of ceremonies at pageants and film commercials. I drove from Tulsa to Oklahoma City each Wednesday to do television commercials for John A. Brown department stores. Mike Smith of Gelders, Holderby, and Smith Advertising Agency helped me in so many ways for so many years. Mike was responsible for my ad work with Gilt Edge Dairies, John A. Brown, and so many other efforts that benefited my career. In the commercial business, I was earning more in a few days a month than I could as a teacher, so I talked myself out of getting a fulltime job of any kind even though that would have given me a greater sense of community.

After each short term project, I slid back into my sad life, with soap operas and slippers. I hated housework, but I loved houses. I thought if we ever settled in the right house in the right neighborhood, then my life would work because I would belong. After a few years, two of my best friends, Beverly Drew Hoster and Annie Arganbright Running, moved to Tulsa. Their presence helped a lot, but could not fill the void in my life.

Nothing went right. I was a desperate housewife. Paul and I fought constantly about everything—money, time, priorities, everything. This was not the kind of marriage I wanted. He was never home. We had no life together. But I did not believe in divorce, regardless of the circumstances. I continued to vacillate between hope and depression.

DR. ROBERT PIERSON

~ ~ ~ *"Jane was not only an example of a devout Christian following Jesus, but also an example of a woman who faced some unusual, painful times and handled herself in a way that clearly showed the power of God in her life. She followed the example of Jesus in finding victory despite the difficulty."*

JEANIE COOPER SHOLER

~ ~ ~ *"I met Jane when were both in a musical at Lyric Theater. She was lovely, talented, and genuine. We have shared joys, sorrows, losses, and laughs. Above all, Jane is a true Christian and an inspiration to us all. She is my daughter's godmother. She has enriched my life and lives of so many others."*

GOVERNOR GEORGE NIGH

~ ~ ~ *"I could be accused of being prejudiced in my comments about Jane because her family ran my campaigns for governor in Laverne. However, it is apparent to all Oklahomans that Jane is an incredible role model. She has brought honor to the state from the day she won the Miss America crown to the present time. Her deep involvement in so many worthy causes is an invaluable asset to Oklahoma."*

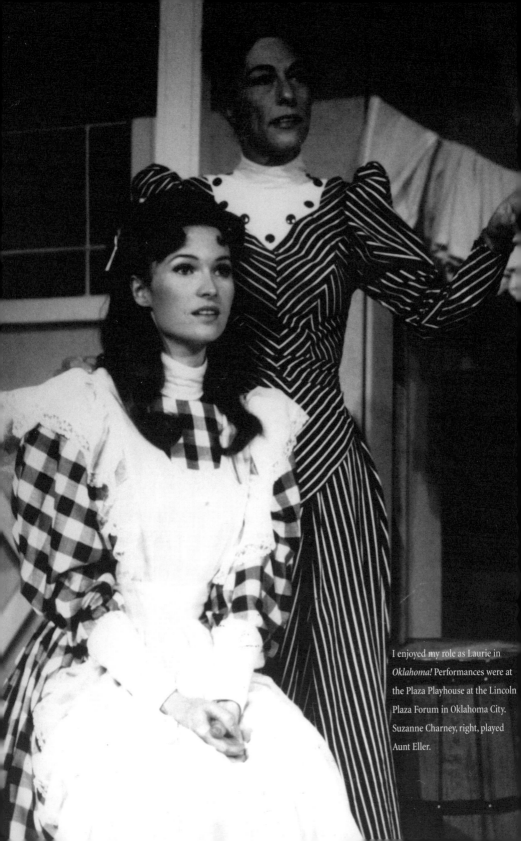

I enjoyed my role as Laurie in *Oklahoma!* Performances were at the Plaza Playhouse at the Lincoln Plaza Forum in Oklahoma City. Suzanne Charney, right, played Aunt Eller.

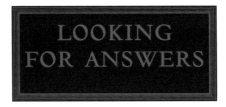

14

LOOKING FOR ANSWERS

round the first of April, 1973, I received a telephone call from Anita Bryant and her husband, Bob Green. Anita had been Miss Oklahoma and runner-up to Miss America. We had several mutual friends and had gotten together once when we were all in Dallas.

Bob had founded a talent agency for Christian speakers and singers called Fishers of Men. He wanted me to speak and give a religious "witness" testimony at a Youth for Christ banquet. He was so enthusiastic, and Paul fully supported the idea. But every time I thought of getting in front of the audience, I felt sick. I had no idea what I could give witness to. My life was a mess behind the scenes.

I began trying to write what my faith was. I had appeared at religious meetings before, but was terribly uncomfortable. I could easily give God all the glory for all the good things in my life, but I was so empty inside and my marriage was anything but fulfilling. When I had sung for Baptist revival meetings with Reverend Boyce Evans, I had felt so guilty that I raised my hand as a sinner who needed to be saved. That was bad, because I was supposed to sing during the invitational when Reverend Evans invited the sinners to the altar.

I considered myself a Christian. I had accepted Jesus Christ as my savior and repented of my sins. That alone had not fixed my life, even if it had assured me of salvation. I was definitely a work in progress. Whenever I tried to express anything about my faith, I became so emotional it left me confused and sad. To me church was a place where I learned to be in front of people, where I felt music was a gift to me, and one to be shared and nurtured. It was a place where I had friends and felt secure and learned to care for others. Church was certainly where God had found me and loved me, but I was on a path with more questions than answers. Now, I know that during that struggling part of my life, I was working out my faith journey. It was no time for me to give witness to anything but God's grace and sing "Jesus loves me, this I know!"

I knew that was not what Fishers of Men had in mind. They wanted a dynamic got-all-the-answers-because-Jesus-is-in-my-life kind of witness. I did not know how to do that without being a hypocrite. To my relief, the Youth for Christ invitation fell through. But my call from Anita and Bob started me reading everything I could get my hands on. There had to be something more to Christianity!

I began regularly attending Christ Methodist Church, pastored by Reverend Bob Pierson. Every word began to be relevant and exciting. I could not believe that all those words, songs, and prayers had been around me my entire life and had little meaning. Now they meant everything! All that time in church growing up had prepared the field, but now I was hearing God's word as if it was being planted in my heart.

I started a diary because I felt reborn. I wanted to record this important personal journey on which I had begun. I wanted to buy into a set of rules, something to make up for a sick marriage, something to hang ambitions on. I wanted to experience religion that would change my life and supply all the answers. And, I wanted it now!

I continued with musical theater. My role as Laurie in *Oklahoma!* with Jim Henline at a new dinner theater at the Lincoln Plaza in Oklahoma City did wonders for my disposition. Paul was supportive. All at once, my career was enjoying a lift, but he thought he was at a dead end without pursuing a master's degree in tax law. His solution was for us to move to New York City and him to attend New York University.

He was shocked at how strongly I reacted to the idea. There was no way I was moving to Manhattan. I had lived a year at the Barclay Hotel with limousines and an expense account. The idea of living in the most expensive place in America on a graduate fellowship in a tiny apartment, without being able to travel much to see my parents, or to attend theater and eat at

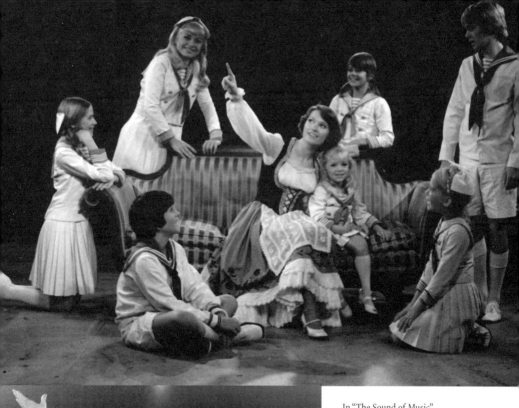

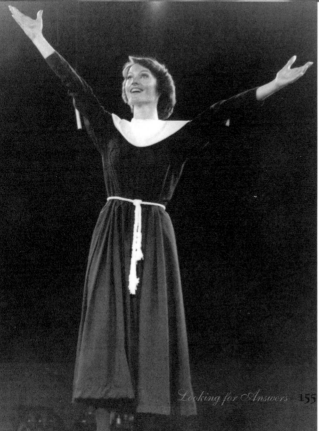

In "The Sound of Music" production in Dallas, Lisa Whelchel, second from right, played one of the Von Trapp children. Lisa later became a major television star in "Facts of Life."

I appeared in the lead role of Maria in "The Sound of Music" at the Crystal Palace Dinner Theater in Dallas in 1974. Buff Shurr directed and choreographed the production.

nice restaurants, was totally unacceptable. I was not paying for another graduate degree, especially in New York City.

Paul compromised and decided to pursue his master's degree at Southern Methodist University (SMU) in Dallas. That was fine with me. I had relatives in Dallas and loved the city.

Living in Dallas was fun with Aunt Honore and two cousins, Mary and Melinda, around to enjoy. Having forced myself to audition for musical theater in Oklahoma City made it easier to audition in Dallas. I was chosen to play Maria in *The Sound of Music* at a new dinner theater. Yvonne de Carlo was the big name as "Elsa," but Maria was the role I wanted and loved.

It was hard work, with only two weeks of rehearsal and six weeks of eight shows a week. As Maria, I was on stage all the time. In between, I was dashing up and down three flights of stairs to change costumes and be in place for the next scene. As a result, I was in great physical shape. I loved every note of every song of every show!

Before the first semester at SMU was completed, Paul concluded he had made a mistake about an advanced degree in tax law. He wanted to move back to Tulsa. I had mixed emotions. But I reasoned that if we returned to Tulsa, I would find some way to have a baby. If I could not have a baby, maybe we could consider adoption.

Going back to Tulsa was even worse than before. We moved into a downtown apartment and Paul was shuttled into a less prestigious position at his law firm. He grew increasingly frustrated with his job.

My reaction was desperation as I saw the walls closing in again. Each day as evening approached and darkness filled the city, I would look out of our 12th floor apartment window and cry with pain. And when the meal I prepared remained in the pots and pans on the stove, finally to be eaten my me, alone, I wanted to scream out, "No! It can't happen again. Please, God, I don't want to live alone as a married person! Help!"

Along came Marabel Morgan's book, *Total Woman*. Through my relationship with Bob Green and Anita Bryant, I was asked to tape a national television commercial for the book. They wanted me to read the book, and if it was something I felt good about, to do a commercial as the spokesperson.

When I hung up the phone, tears of joy filled my eyes. God had answered my prayer—a miracle had happened—it was another example of God's grace being poured out on me. I was somebody—needed and wanted.

I raced to the nearest bookstore and purchased a copy of *Total Woman*. It was urgent that I read it, believe it, practice it immediately, so I could testify to its benefits. When I arrived at the apartment, I took a diet drink from the refrigerator and curled up in a chair with the book. I began underlining almost every sentence. I believed! I believed!

For example, part of our problem was that Paul worked late almost every weeknight and every weekend. I blamed him because we had no fun in our life together. The book said it was because the wife nags. The author was right—I complained too much. Or, in the gospel according to Marabel, husbands stay at work because their wives were not exciting enough. She was right again—I felt about as exciting as an empty box.

I read the book and reread it. I wanted desperately to be a total woman and be a religious, submissive wife. I kept trying hard to make my marriage work.

But after only a few weeks, I had to admit to myself that my marriage was still grossly unhappy, so I turned down the opportunity to be the spokesperson for the book. I could not embarrass myself by talking about marital bliss. The conflicts between Paul and me were far beyond solving with simple answers.

One positive result of me reading the book was that I was convinced that I needed to take control of my own life. I decided to return to school for a masters of arts degree in humanities at the University of Tulsa. God gave me a wonderful counselor, Kara Gay Neal. As part of the requisites for the advanced degree, I had to take a women's history seminar.

I knew little about the women's movement. I had always thought that women activists were radical, attention-seeking, jealous women who burned their bras in Atlantic City. Nothing prepared me for what I was learning. I discovered that the lonely path I was traveling was crowded with all kinds of other women.

For example, in 1770 Abigail Adams wrote to her husband, who would become our second president, pleading for women's rights:

Remember the ladies and be more generous and favorable to them than were your ancestors. Do not put such unlimited power into the hands of husbands. Remember all men would be tyrants if they could. If particular care and attention are not paid to the ladies, we are determined to foment a rebellion and will not hold ourselves bound to obey any laws, in which we have no voice or representation.

Abigail Adams did not act on her threats, but years later other women did. In 1848, the first women's rights convention was held in Seneca Falls, New York. Women like Lucretia Mott and Elizabeth Cady Stanton took on the task of personhood for women. They began a movement that would eventually result in the right to vote for women and arguments for equal pay and equal status with American men.

With support from my local church, Christ United Methodist Church, in Tulsa, I began to develop a new concept of self-awareness. A Christian commitment that I had been working so hard to experience did happen, not as a flash of lightning, but as a glow that was nurtured by a community of caring people who offered to share my life without intruding. I attended church regularly, volunteered as the church receptionist, was part of many small groups, and soaked up the love and support they offered.

It was an important commitment in my life to become a part of the church on my own. I would desperately need the chuch, because, as incredible as it seemed, in the midst of everything else, I was pregnant!

I had wanted a baby from the first day of our marriage. One of the reasons I had worked so hard at our marriage was my deep desire to have children. Every person I had ever dated back to high school had been subconsciously evaluated as a future father. What would our children look like and be like? What names would go well with their last name?

Getting pregnant had not been easy for me. I went without birth control for years, but never got pregnant. I began reading books about fertility drugs and procedures. After I broached the subject of adoption, I looked further into medical treatment to help me get pregnant. I knew having a baby would surely help our marriage, so I underwent a procedure to clear a partial blockage of one of my tubes.

When I walked out of the doctor's office in November, 1975, with news I was pregnant, I was on top of the world. Paul and I were both in disbelief for days because it had been so hard to get pregnant.

Soon after the news, I was a mistress of ceremonies at the OU Homecoming Show at the Lloyd Noble Center in Norman with Bob Hope, Phyllis Diller, and the New Christy Minstrels. I had to work out several jokes with Bob. He did not give you a lot of preparation time to be his partner, but I somehow pulled it off. He was a hero!

I remember waiting in my dressing room and looking at myself in the mirror. Other than Paul, no one knew of my special secret. A baby—the most important thing that would ever happen to me—God's greatest gift!

Back in Tulsa, I watched my stomach every day—while I was walking I would notice my weirdly shaped shadow. Spring was never so beautiful!

I sat most of June on the sofa in front of a fan. I was fat and hot. The day before my son was born, a lady who lived in our neighborhood called because our yard did not look nice. She angrily reminded me that I had been Miss America and she could not believe I would be so unpatriotic as not to have my yard beautiful for the Bicentennial celebration. Her anger threw me into two hours of crying. I was so scared about childbirth, our marriage, and keeping my house and myself together.

The situation between Paul and me was not made better by pregnancy. In fact, I had considered moving to Oklahoma City several times during the spring. But I believed that a baby would make a huge difference in my relationship with Paul. I did not want to live alone and change doctors during the pregnancy. Instead of moving, I yelled, screamed, cried, and threatened, but I stayed.

On Sunday morning, July 4, 1976, on America's 200th birthday, Tyler Jayroe Petersen was born. I had my first labor pains at 2:00 a.m. and went to the hospital four hours later. After 14 hours of unproductive labor, the doctor performed a C-Section. Tyler weighed nine pounds. Giving birth to such a beautiful little boy was a great celebration! Toni Spencer called him "Yankee Doodle!"

On the day I brought Tyler home, Paul was out of town. I could hardly get out of bed with my incision from the C-Section. My mother, who had stayed with me for several days, had to go home. Tyler had colic and I was fighting a bladder infection. I was angry, confused, frustrated, and scared. I believe Paul had left our marriage emotionally a long time before, but he had trouble knowing how to leave it physically. There were so many times

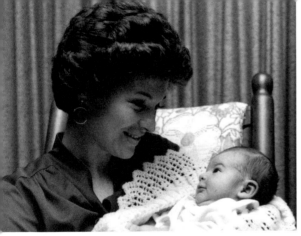

My darling son, Tyler Jayroe Petersen, was born on July 4, 1976, America's 200th birthday.

that I was alone and had no idea where he was. I was embarrassed and my pride prevented me from telling my friends how bad the situation really was.

Loneliness was overwhelming. One night, I was alone with my crying baby and I had a burning 104-degree fever. I had to make a decision. I had to leave, but even when I told Paul we were separating, I was bluffing. I still believed if I threatened to leave, he would change. Instead, he agreed to the separation. On our eighth anniversary, August 16, 1976, my parents moved me out.

I had no idea what I was in for. If I had been healthy and had all my wits about me, maybe it would have been easier. Instead, I was a new mother and was physically and emotionally down. The next few months were pure hell! I left the house and Tyler's baby room that I had worked so hard on. I left my church, my friends, my identity. I took my clothes, my tears, my dog, and my baby, and headed to Oklahoma City to live with my sister. There, I found incredible support and encouragement. Don and Judy always made me feel welcome. They moved my nephew out of his bedroom, moved the baby bed in, and I started trying to survive minute-by-minute.

I had no idea how long I would be anywhere. But the more distance I placed between me and my former life, the more I knew in my heart that I could not return. I had to make a new start, not from the bottom, but from near the bottom. Surely no one ever had more self-pity and felt more abused and taken advantage of. Right or wrong, that was the runway that now stretched before me.

Jane Jayroe, former wife, former Miss America, former something, now new mother and single parent, was starting over.

DR. NORMAN NEAVES

~ ~ ~ *"Jane is a tribute to her father and mother, the people of
Oklahoma who have been "her people," and to the people of
America. She knows real grace is always simple grace and that
grace has the inherent gift of mixing the ordinary and
extraordinary, the plain and the sophisticated, the common and
the exception. There are few people in this world who have the
ability to bring that kind of grace into the world as beautifully
and as genuinely as does Jane."*

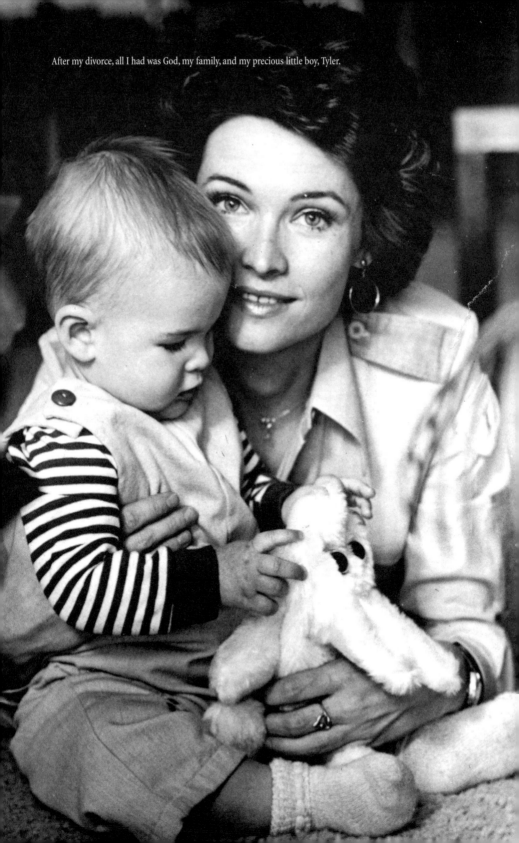

After my divorce, all I had was God, my family, and my precious little boy, Tyler.

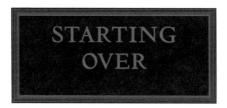

15

STARTING OVER

*S*eparation was like my first day back at the Student Union cafeteria at OCU after spending a year as Miss America. It felt like everyone was looking at me.

With all the events going on in the world, I could not conceive that my marital problems were important to others. Yet a few days after I moved in with my sister, a newspaper ran a front page story about my separation and impending divorce. I was in bed when Judy brought me the paper. I wanted to stay in bed and pull the covers over my head forever. Regardless of the benign contents of the newspaper article, the headline shouted to me, "Jane Jayroe, big disappointment, fails at marriage!" Not only did I feel like a failure, I felt as if I had let the entire state of Oklahoma down.

As a child, I learned the 23rd Psalm, and remembered the words, "in the valley of shadow of death." That is where I was in 1976. I felt like death, although I was alive and responsible for a tiny baby boy. Nine years after being Miss America, eight years after a happily-ever-after wedding, three weeks after a baby boy was born on the Fourth of July, I was at the bottom of the barrel.

I had no job, no money, no self-confidence, and no home. After being Miss America I had been offered several high paying jobs, but turned them down to concentrate on getting married. I had put all my eggs in one basket—a husband—and the basket broke and Jane came tumbling down.

God's grace was all I had—and His grace was more than sufficient for me, although it was not a speedy turn around. It was a plodding kind of recovery, one foot in front of the other. Grit is what matters when things go south in life. To quote Winston Churchill, "Never, ever give up!"

News reporters began calling me, but I did not know what to say. I would have liked answers to some of the same questions—what was I going to do? Who would take care of my son and me? Where would we live? Was I going to work? Were there any special plans? On and on the questions went—but there were no answers.

Despite how difficult the separation was, it did help me face the inevitable—my marriage in Camelot not only had never been, but would never be. Blame and anger were useless, although I wasted a lot of emotional strength blaming Paul and being hurt and enraged. I had no goals, no plans, no dreams. My body still carried the effects of pregnancy. I felt fat, unpretty, unwanted, and I was totally unhappy. But, I had to get on with my life. My little boy deserved better than a depressed, brooding mother sitting at home with no purpose in life.

What I had to fight was the magnetic quality of the giant hole of depression in which I found myself. It was not like a hole that one would leap into, but was like a spiral tube with smooth sides—I could not hang on nor go back up. Once in awhile, I felt like I could spread my arms and "get a grip" on the sides of the tube, but then something else would happen and I would again start the downward fall. What if there was no bottom? How could I keep functioning?

In the spiraling down of that darkness, I finally had the courage to let go. I fell, crying and hurting, into the cushion of God's grace and love. God's presence began lifting me up—not all at once—there was no bold stroke of healing. But there were small steps that would lead me to the top and solid ground.

When God calmed my insides a little, I began seeing ways to help myself. I asked for help from my family, friends, and church. I enrolled in an exercise program at church. The jumping around to music helped my body and my mind. I planned ahead to get through the loneliest times of the week. Sunday nights became my toughest times.

With my mind operating more clearly, I realized that God was with me every step of the way. Life was tougher than I had thought, and certainly more unfair. But I found God to be bigger than I thought and more personally loving to me. I could see light at the end of the tunnel—and it was not a train coming at me!

I made a big emotional step when I decided to move from my sister's home. We had been an interruption in their lives, but I could not bear to even think of moving out for a long time.

When our house in Tulsa sold, I found a duplex a few blocks from Judy and Don and my closest friend, Kerry Robertson. It was being leased by some of Judy's friends to temporarily store their furniture. They generously offered to let me stay there, but it was a depressing option for me. It was just not a space that reflected my needs or desires. But as the saying goes, "beggars can't be choosers!" and I was tying to be practical. The duplex was crowded and gloomy, with no back yard for Bartok, my faithful dog.

So, in the middle of one night, Paul brought the rest of my personal belongings from Tulsa and put them in the garage in the duplex. I now had a new address, a new phone number, and a new existence.

The very next week, my luck changed. The duplex next door became available. It was light and airy. Even though it meant more rent, I committed, signed the lease, and Tyler and I moved in. It was much smaller than any home Paul and I had lived in, but I was humbled. It was so welcome!

The numbness of my plight was wearing off and I began to think about the future. My most obvious need was money. My parents were more than willing to help, but they were nearing retirement and had carefully planned and saved just for their living. As I lay awake at night, I was worried I could not pay the bills or make it on my own. What was I to do? Did I want to be teacher? A nurse? How would I leave my baby while I was working?

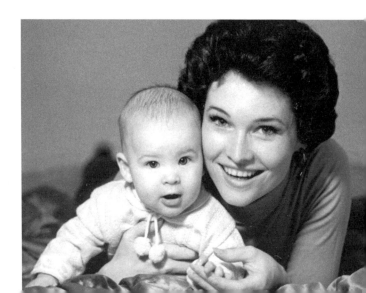

Even after I began working, I could not wait to come home at night and spend time with Tyler. Courtesy J.W. Robertson.

A huge bright spot in my shattered life was Tyler, my healthy baby boy who demanded center stage. Nothing felt more intense than the joy of picking him up in the morning or laughing at him laugh at me. I found his behavior fascinating, incredible, and fun.

With only the two of us in the duplex, I had trouble figuring out how to do anything. I tried to take showers and do laundry when he was asleep. If he was awake, it was impossible to take a shower. I tried that once, but he emptied a giant economy size bottle of shampoo on the carpet.

By January 11, 1977, there was a glimmer of hope in my future. The holidays had been tough, but I found the new year bright. I wrote in my journal: "It doesn't hurt anymore. Was there security in the pain? Am I pushed into a more responsible arena now? Time to grow up and continue. I feel like a bird. I was prematurely let out of a nest because I appeared to be ready to fly beautifully (Miss America). Instead I flew as a response to the wind and elements, constantly afraid of falling and constantly seeking to find a way back. I flew high and I learned a lot but was afraid to look down. Then I found another nest (marriage). Regardless of how it was built and rebuilt, it could not hold together. When it broke, it fell. On the way down, I discovered how to fly, now I feel movement around me as I soar and glide and dive. It feels so good. I may find a direction and somewhere to go or I may find a lack of direction worthwhile."

In retrospect, there were some real principles that pulled me up and taught me to fly. It just takes time to heal. I can vividly remember my friend, Sue Wells, who had gone through a divorce, telling me, "One day, you won't even know it, but you will look up and the pain will be gone!" Maybe that was obvious to everyone but me.

Friends like Sue and Kerry helped me put my life together. They made my 30th birthday special, when I looked and felt like I was 50. They shared the tears and helped me laugh. How great it felt to laugh again!

It was the same with my newly divorced friend, Jeannie Cooper. We sat at her parent's table on New Year's Day and laughed like crazy as we ate our black eyed peas, hoping for a better year.

I decided to go back to school to finish my masters degree in humanities. Dr. Ann Carlton taught a literature class at OCU and was my advisor. She guided me through a maze of classics such as Little Women and Scarlet

Letter. I realized that even though I was alone, I was becoming happy, self-directed, and involved in life.

I identified with Kate Chopin's novel, *The Awakening*. I could not believe a book written in 1899 could have such relevance in my life in 1977. She wrote: "Perhaps it is better to wake up after all, even to suffer rather than to remain a dupe to illusion all one's life. I would give up the unessential; I would give my money, I would give my life for my children; but I would not give myself. I can't make it more clear; it's only something which I am beginning to comprehend, which is revealing itself to me."

Classes at my church, Church of the Servant, helped me feel like I belonged. That warm feeling also helped me forgive myself for my mistakes and reach out to others who were hurting. What a blessing it was to share my feelings and God's promises with another person who was going through a difficult time. Dr. Norman Neaves and his wife, Kip, were among the most important people in my life. They were so loving and sensitive to my pain. I cannot imagine my life without them.

When I first walked into the foyer at Church of the Servant on Northwest Expressway in Oklahoma City, I knew it was the place for me. In the middle of the greeting area was an old beat-up garbage can with flowers growing from it. That was my life—a mess. I felt all dented but I believed God could redeem any situation—even mine. This would be my church home, and the possibility of flowers blooming again in the garbage can that life can sometimes be, brought tears to me eyes and hope to my heart.

A nice career boost came in August, 1977. I was paired with the legendary Art Linkletter to host a 12-program television series for volunteer teachers. Produced by the Oklahoma Educational Television Authority (OETA), the programs were syndicated nationwide.

With the help of my father, I found a regular job as an arts-in-education specialist at the Oklahoma State Department of Education. With my masters degree and good grades on my transcript, I moved into the job, with excitement about the promotion of arts throughout the education system. My immediate boss, Peggy Long, became one of my best friends and a terrific role model. She was also divorced and was doing a wonderful job of raising her daughter. She taught me a lot about work and life, as did her colleague, Charles Moore, who was also a single parent and an A-plus person.

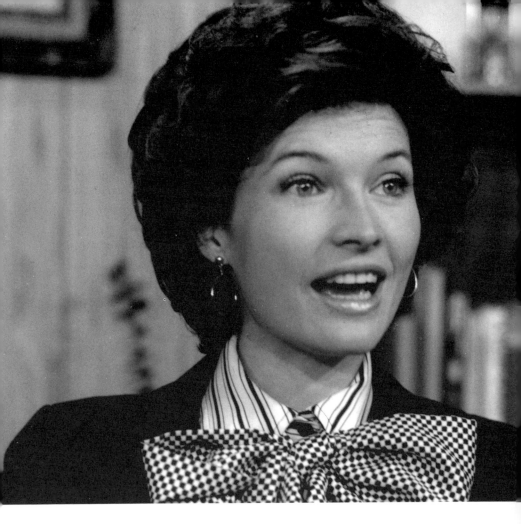

Above, hosting a television show for the State Department of Education was great training for my future television career. Bottom right, I learned a lot from the great Art Linkletter, seated with me in the photo at right, when I co-hosted a series of television shows for volunteer teachers. Top right, when Tyler and I moved into a home in the Surrey Hills section of northwest Oklahoma City, we had plenty of space for riding a bicycle. Courtesy Oklahoma Publishing Company. Right, a newspaper cartoonist's version of a beauty queen, with crown, as a television newscaster.

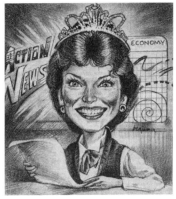

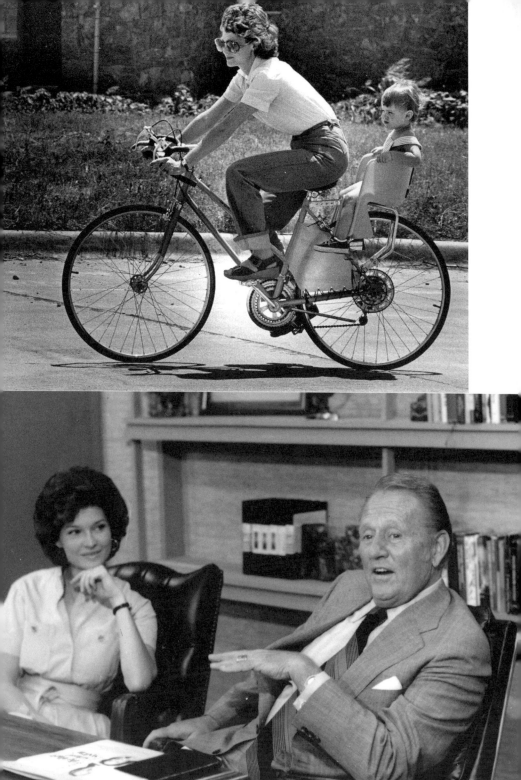

I was worried about someone keeping Tyler, but was blessed with a family across the street from Kerry Robertson. Jesse, Vileta, Pam, and Debbie Terpening adopted Tyler and me as their own. Vileta was another mother to my son and everyone in the family loved him. Being away from Tyler during the day made me realize he was the best thing I had ever done in life. He brought such joy to me—and always has.

In my job at the Department of Education, I produced and hosted a 30-minute public service program that I mistakenly thought no one ever watched. It was invaluable training for an unexpected opportunity that was headed my way.

In 1977, I received a call from Foster Morgan, the news director at KOCO-TV, Channel 5, in Oklahoma City. The ABC affiliate was interested in hiring a female co-anchor for the local evening news. At that time, female anchors during prime time were so new that the primary concern was to hire someone who would look good on the air. There were few women in the newsroom at Channel 5, and none on the air in an anchor role.

I had no prior experience as a journalist but was excited about this new challenge. I did not have a journalism degree, but I did have vast experience in communicating under stress. That was one of the gifts learned as Miss America. I had to speak hundreds of times, to young and old alike. At the time, I had no idea that the stressful year as Miss America was preparing me for a job as a television news anchor.

I felt good about the audition in which I was asked to take wire copy and write a portion of a newscast. Again, my bachelor's degree in music education and master of arts from Tulsa University served me well.

After the audition, General Manager Al Parsons offered me $25,000 a year to be the co-anchor on the 6:00 p.m. and 10:00 p.m. newscasts. The salary was almost twice what I was making at the Department of Education. Even though I would surely endure criticism for not being a trained journalist, I was ready to tackle the new job. The only downside, as a single mom, was the prospect of being away from Tyler during the evening hours.

I was jumping back in the fish bowl without the protection of the Miss America organization. But I had no illusions about the new job—I knew it be would be hard work in a fast paced industry that was in the midst of fundamental change.

BILL GEDDIE

~ ~ ~ *"Jane came into my life in my first year of television. The fact that I would be working with someone who most people in Oklahoma knew was very exciting. It was less exciting for the old hands at KOCO-TV. For them, she represented all that was going to hell in a hand basket about television news. She was not a trained journalist and, worst of all for some of them, she was a former Miss America. But Jane never pretended to be anything other than what she was. She asked questions, deferred to the news pros in the office, and was always kind and cordial."*

BARBARA GEDDIE

~ ~ ~ *"I was a news producer when Jane first came to KOCO-TV. Bill, not yet my husband, worked as a news cameraman. Television news was in a state of flux and change. It was being transformed from public service news into a lucrative news business. It was researched by consultants, scrutinized by focus groups, formatted, and marketed to reflect a news "show" that would draw local sponsors.*
Jane was part of a new wave of employees being introduced to the mindset of how news would change to compliment new technology. She approached the job from the get-go with poise and ease."

KAREN HUGHES

~ ~ ~ *"I admired Jane's grace and strength during our years at KXAS-TV. I am thankful for her wonderful example and witness."*

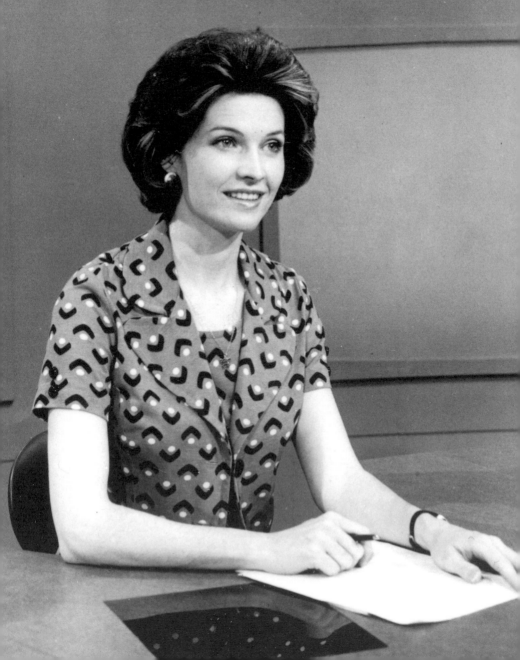

I was comfortable most of the time on the news set at KOCO-TV in Oklahoma City.

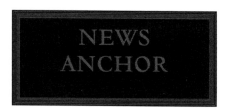

16

NEWS ANCHOR

I had it all! My 18-month-old baby, Tyler, was the greatest thing that ever happened to me, and I loved my job as co-anchor of KOCO-TV's 5 Alive News Center. I was honored to be one of the few women newscasters on television—I was plowing new ground.

There was no one at the television station to train someone who had never worked a day in the news business—so I trained myself. I practiced and practiced writing copy. For the month before I went on the air, I rehearsed in front of the mirror at home. We had only one full run through with almost an entire new on-camera group before actually going on the air.

I became accustomed to cues from floor crews, talking into a camera with a tiny light, and ignoring the activity behind the cameras as technical people moved cables and set up new shots.

I enjoyed not only the on-camera work, but the writing, producing, and editing. It was fulfilling to be on a "team" with photographers, assignment editors, producers, and reporters. I loved doing something that mattered. I cherished being a part of the lives of people of Oklahoma. It was incredible to watch the process of communication that traveled from a cold room with three cameras, a flimsy news desk, and a hundred lights, through the camera lens into homes in Oklahoma.

At first, media types were critical that someone with no background in journalism could become an instant on-the-air news journalist. Newspaper reviewers hung me out to dry, calling me a beauty queen, not a journalist. In a column titled "Jive Alive," Chan Lowe in *The Daily Oklahoman*, came

It takes a lot of people to produce daily news and sports shows at a major television station. This was the KOCO-TV family in 1978. Front row, left to right, General De Hong, Ivy Thorpe, Chris Sloat, Patty Green, Scott Massey, and Ann Dee Lee. Second row, Rick Thompson, Chess Rutledge, Gan Matthews, Chris Lee, John Dumontel, Paula McCarter, and Kevin Kerringan. Back row, Tony Sellers, Ed "Ho Ho" Birchall, Vince Orza, Wayne Shattuck, Jack Bowen, me, Karim E. Karim, Rick Buchanan, Joyce Jackson, Ron Stahl, Dennis Gimmel.

down heavy on Channel 5 for confusing journalism and entertainment.

However, just a few months later, Chan apologized in his column. He wrote, "As it turns out, Miss Jayroe is one of the few bright spots of that program, showing an aptitude for news coverage and anchoring which more than vindicate her." Chan also said I was the "backbone" of the newscasts at Channel 5.

I was fairly confident of my ability as a communicator as long as I could read copy I had written. However, I was less than confident about ad-libbing into weather or sports segments. I had reason to be concerned. On a March evening when the threat of severe weather in Oklahoma might keep viewers up past their bedtime, I turned to weatherman Wayne Shattuck, our new good-looking, young meteorologist, and said, "Shall we go to bed now, or stay up awhile?"

I am not sure what I said after that, but everyone in the studio, including my co-anchor and sportscasters, were rolling with laughter. Wayne went right on. I blushed and became totally incapacitated. What had I gotten myself into now?

The experience with my first two co-anchors at Channel 5 was not good. The first one was offended that he was teamed with a non-journalist. He told others he feared he would have to write all the copy. At least his resignation was innovative—he took a 45 rpm record of the song, "Take This Job and Shove It," signed his name on the label, and hung the record on the news director's door.

The second co-anchor was recruited from out of state, and lasted only a short term. The third co-anchor, Jack Bowen, stuck. Jack taught me many things about news journalism and we worked well together.

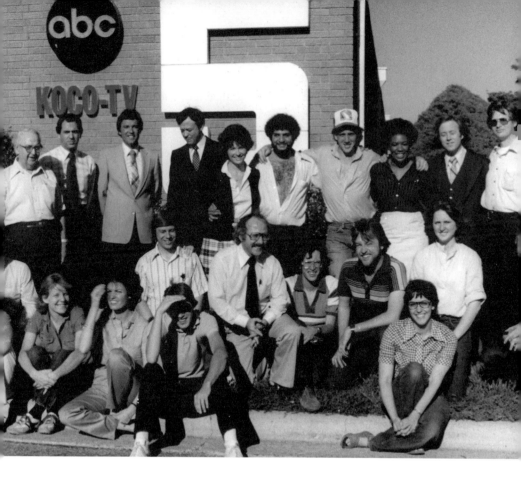

The Channel 5 news team really became successful when Tom Kirby became news director. Tom had been executive producer at KBTV in Denver, Colorado, Channel 5's sister station owned by Combined Communications. Tom's job was difficult. Chan Lowe, in is newspaper column, said, "Kirby is going to need of lot of optimism to tackle the wreckage he is about to inherit."

Tom taught me a lot about television news and anchoring. He worked on my on-air performance, my writing style, and taught me the importance of writing to pictures. Tom was an encourager and helped all of us to believe in ourselves and the importance, and fun, of striving to make every day and every newscast the best we could deliver. And when we did, we received a personal note from Tom with a specific comment about something we did well.

Being on television placed me back in the public spotlight—but it was different this time. I still heard people at the mall or in restaurants say, "Isn't that Jane Jayroe?" But, the recognition was not just for winning one contest or how I looked in a swimsuit or formal gown. The public's recognition was now based upon my performance each night in their home. There was a greater sense of connectedness. The feeling so often was just one of familiarity.

For many years, a plaque that read, "Lord Help Me Survive My Blessings," hung over my sister's sink. Joyfully, that prayer now fit me. I had a wonderful job and career and a bouncing toddler who was the light of my life. At times, the only bumps in my road came from dealing with trivial, and unimportant, jobs such as getting my car repaired, making sure I had enough diapers, trying to get the door to my house open at 11:00 p.m. while holding Tyler and all his stuff, or struggling to keep Bartok, my dog, from barking and jumping and waking Tyler. To keep everything in perspective, I usually turned my exhaustion into laughter.

On a personal level, I met Wayne Robinson, a writer in Oklahoma City who would soon move to California. We fell in love, and believed we could join our two families and have a long-distance marriage. He worked in Los Angeles all week and commuted to Oklahoma City for the weekends.

We were married in 1979 in Carmel, California. I gained a new family, Brett, Laura, and Carol, and now had someone with whom to share responsibility. Wayne was an outstanding father and his children were very special. I met Wayne at an extremely vulnerable time in my life. I wanted so badly to be married and get on with my life and have more children. I wanted help with my life. I really ran ahead of God and my marriage with Wayne never quite worked.

A great tragedy occurred on January 18, 1980. On his way home from work, Judy's husband, Don, pulled over on the side of the road and died of a heart attack. He was only 42 years old. The authorities came to me and I rushed home from the station to be with my sister, only to find out she had not yet been told of Don's death. I thought maybe it was a bad dream. It was not!

Judy braved the storm of a tragic loss and went on to do a stellar job of raising their three sons, Jace, Dal, and Cade. After Don's funeral, Judy

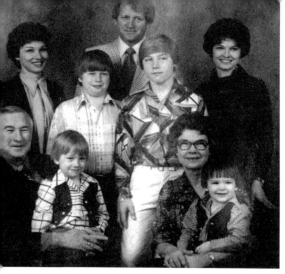

By the time I became a television news anchor, the Jayroe family was growing. Sitting, left to right, Daddy, Cade Wieser, Mother, and Tyler Jayroe. Standing, Judy Jayroe Wieser, Dal Wieser, Don Wieser, Jace Wieser, and me. Don died suddenly in 1980. Several years later, Judy married Frank Elmore from the Laverne area. Frank and his daughters, Kathy and Tanya, have enriched our family in every way. Would you believe they love basketball and Frank's grandson, Austin Johnson, plays for the OU Sooners.

returned to teaching music at Yukon, Oklahoma. Her star senior student and one of Don's football players came to see Judy and sang her a song he had written, "Don't Worry, We'll Take of Your Woman." The student was Garth Brooks.

In 1980, after nearly two years on the air, I began receiving job offers from around the nation. I was interested in only one—in the Dallas-Fort Worth television market. I did not apply for a job in the market, but when KXAS-TV called, I agreed to audition. I did not want to leave my family and friends in Oklahoma, especially Judy, but moving into a top ten television market would be great for my career, and would significantly increase my salary.

In April, 1980, I made the official announcement that I was leaving Channel 5 for KXAS-TV. *The Daily Oklahoman* was very kind in saying that Channel 5 would miss me. The newspaper gave me much of the credit for the resurrection of Channel 5's ratings during the local news blocks.

My departure caused Channel 5's ownership to sue KXAS-TV, seeking a court order to prevent the Texas station from trying to hire other anchors from Channel 5. I had a clause in my contract with Channel 5 that I could leave anytime if given an opportunity at a top ten national market. Dallas-Fort Worth fit that description, but the contracts of other anchors at the station, such as Jack Bowen, did not contain such provisions. To prevent more litigation, KXAS agreed not to talk to Jack or anyone else under contract at Channel 5.

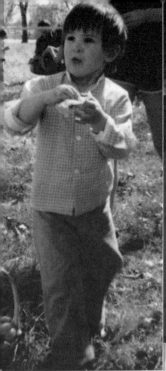

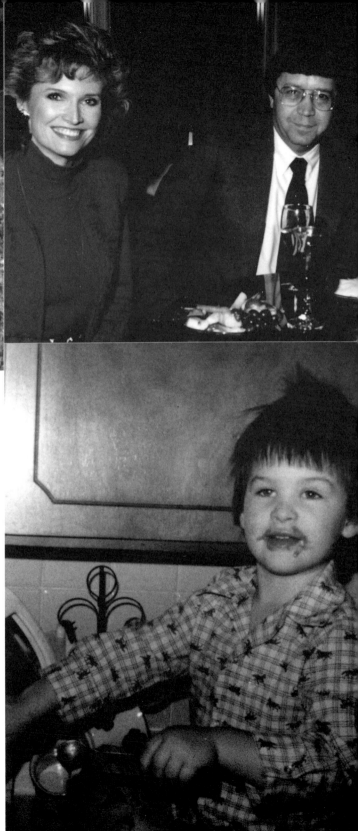

Above, Tyler was such a fun little guy. We had a wonderful relationship in spite of some difficult circumstances. Right, Tyler was happiest when he "helped" his Grandmother Lene in the kitchen. Above right, my great friend at KOCO-TV was news director Tom Kirby who later became general manager of the television station.

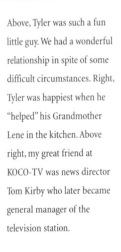

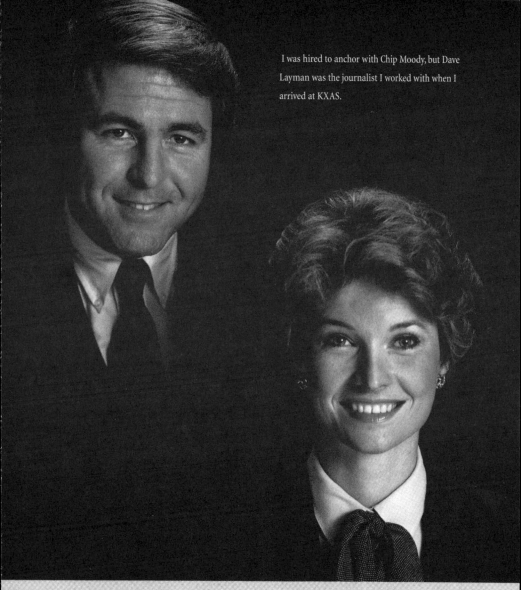

I was hired to anchor with Chip Moody, but Dave Layman was the journalist I worked with when I arrived at KXAS.

These people are getting a reputation.

Dave Layman and Jane Jayroe are becoming Dallas/Fort Worth's most looked-at news team. They're getting a reputation as communicators with a bright, fresh, intelligent style. That's what people are talking about: Dave Layman and Jane Jayroe. They're concerned, honest, down-to-earth journalists with a dedication that makes them worthy of their reputation. Look for them weeknights at 6 and 10, when they give it all they've got!

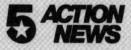

5 ACTION NEWS

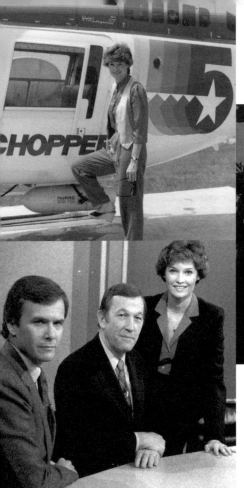

Left, the Channel 5 helicopter often whisked me away to cover news stories in the Dallas-Fort Worth area. Top right, I worked with Scott and Jane Pelley at KXAS. Both were excellent broadcast journalists.

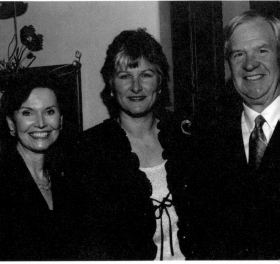

As an NBC affiliate anchor, I met some of the great television journalists of our time. In New York City, I met with NBC's Tom Brokaw, left, and Roger Mudd.

While I was at KXAS, Karen Hughes became an intern in the newsroom. She did well—and later was selected by President George W. Bush as a close campaign and communications advisor. The photograph above was taken when she came to Oklahoma City University as the keynote speaker for a conference. Bottom right, I was honored to be voted the top female news anchor in the Dallas-Fort Worth market, one of the top ten television markets in the nation. I was a member of a great team—Left to right, Brad Wright, Scott Murray, and Harold Taft, a graduate of Oklahoma's Phillips University in Enid, who became a pioneer television meteorologist. He was among the first television weathermen to use radar.

I walked into a hornet's nest at KXAS, the NBC affiliate in the Dallas-Fort Worth metroplex. I was greeted with a headline in the *Dallas Morning News*, "KXAS inherits Barbie doll beauty for news." The headline did not hurt my feelings—it just made me want to prove that I was now a real television newscaster and had worked hard in Oklahoma City to learn the business.

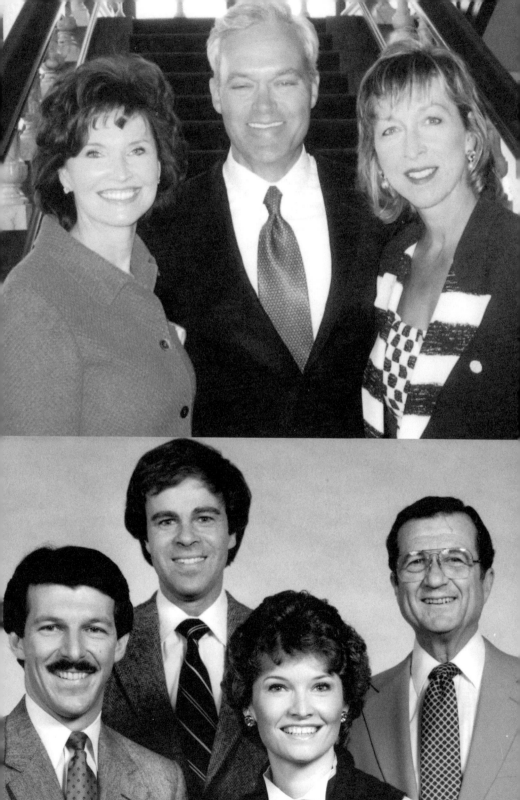

By 1980, KXAS, once the pillar of local news, had plummeted to the bottom in ratings. Heads began to roll and a new face, mine, was added to the 6:00 p.m. and 10:00 p.m. news shows. The station's biggest asset was Chip Moody, a veteran anchorman with whom I was to join forces. He had good looks, excellent skills, and a Texas-sounding voice. He also was one of the best anchors in the market.

Chip was wanting a co-anchor—he had expressed openly his disdain for having to write and deliver the entire newscast alone. However, just before I arrived in May, Chip had been talking to officials of KXAS' competition, KDFW, Channel 4. He shocked his colleagues by announcing he was leaving KXAS. So, my co-anchor was gone before I ever got a chance to work with him. Chip later said that my arrival had nothing to do with him leaving.

I was under tremendous pressure from the day I arrived at KXAS-TV. I was aware of what the *Dallas Morning News* called "the oppressive weight of a floundering news department" on my "slender shoulders."

I tried very hard to make a good impression and to take advantage of the opportunity to deliver the news in one of the nation's largest markets. I wrote my own copy, wore very little makeup, and prayed a little before my first newscast. A reporter saw my determination and wrote:

The day of her first on-air appearance, she emerged from the grimy little newsroom bathroom, and the transformation was startling. Her makeup was perfect, and her eyes had a determined glint. Jane Jayroe looked the part. A veteran photographer stared in amazement, "She cleans up read good, don't she?" he muttered.

Wayne and I moved into a home just a few blocks from the KXAS studio in Fort Worth. He gave up a lucrative job in California for us to be able to live together. The move also put him closer to his children. We were greeted in Texas with the hottest summer on record. The week I went on the air, Wayne's three children came for the summer just as I prepared to go to Detroit, Michigan, to cover the Republican National Convention. It was difficult, because I did not know one single Republican from Texas at the convention. I had to learn about Texas Republican politics quickly.

I worked with so many true broadcast professionals at KXAS. Harold Taft, a native Oklahoman who was one of the world's most recognized weathermen, was a lovable father image and great mentor. Karen Parfitt, better known as Karen Hughes, a close advisor to President George W. Bush, was first an intern, then a reporter at the station. Even though Karen was just a pup during those days, she impressed everyone with her intellect, energy, and work ethic. I remain a huge fan of Karen Hughes.

Scott Pelley, who married Jane Boone, a KXAS reporter from western Oklahoma, was my news producer at KXAS. He moved on to CBS News, "60 Minutes," and a stunning career. He is one of the finest people I have known. Our news director, Bill Vance, treated me wonderfully. During my first year at KXAS, we began putting together a great team that moved steadily up in the ratings, especially during the 6:00 p.m. time slot. The station began winning awards and our newscasts were gaining respect among viewers and competitors. We were number one in ratings in five of the six daily news shows.

My first co-anchor was Dave Layman, a journalist's journalist and truly great guy. We worked well together. After he left, Brad Wright became my sixth co-anchor in six years of television news. Brad was a dedicated parent, as well as a great news anchor.

To prove that I was serious about broadcast journalism, I did special news reports on the hardest topics I could imagine. I worked with the police sex crimes unit, attended a union meeting when Braniff Airlines was going under, covered tough political and weather stories, and even visited the infamous Dallas County Jail. There was no magic formula for our success—just determination and grit.

The same reporter who called me a "Barbie" when I arrived in Dallas-Fort Worth must have changed his mind. A year later, he chose me as the first journalist to be on the cover of a special feature in his newspaper.

Even in Dallas-Fort Worth, I was still breaking ground as a female anchor. It had always been a male-dominated field. Barbara Walters had done feature stories for NBC's "Today Show" for years, but there were few women in television newsrooms around the country. It changed in a hurry. News directors did not know what to do with women. There was usually no dressing room for a female on-air person. Men slapped powder on as they walked into the studio—it took us girls a little longer to look presentable for the camera.

At KXAS, when the male anchor was gone, the news director always put someone else in his place to co-anchor with me. When I was gone, the male anchor did the news by himself. I pointed that out after awhile, and they let me solo as well. I guess news directors were still not sure how accepting the public was of hearing the hard news of the day from a woman.

The management at KXAS certainly took chances where I was concerned. They taught me—they supported me. After two years in Texas, my salary was doubled and my contract extended. I was always my own agent. It was a win/win professional situation. I was a good fit for the metroplex viewing audience and I enjoyed my work immensely.

My toughest job was still trying to juggle family life and a television career. I went to work at 2:00 p.m., but took off an hour later to pick up Tyler from elementary school. I was almost always able to go home after the 6:00 show before I had to prepare for the late night newscast. Living close to the station was a necessity.

Through Tyler's school, God gave me a wonderful new friend, Sue Sewell. I was always dependent on a good friend for help with school stuff and Tyler. Sue became more than a neighborhood friend—she became a true sister in Christ on a lifelong journey we continue to share.

We were also blessed to find our angel Maria to take care of Tyler. Leaving the Terpening family in Oklahoma City was hard. I tried several childcare situations in Fort Worth that were not what I wanted for my child. Finally, a friend at work mentioned that her Aunt Mary Leos in San Antonio, Texas, might be available to care for Tyler.

The woman who appeared on my doorstep did not match my preconceived image of the ideal nanny. Mary was tiny and older. Her clothes were ragged, mismatched, and held together with safety pins. She was very shy and spoke in broken English. Whatever reservations I had about Mary's ability were erased when Tyler took her by the hand and led her into the house. Mary listened and smiled as Tyler jabbered for the next few hours. They colored and watched television together. There was no doubt that Mary was the perfect nanny for Tyler. She came to live with us when Tyler was four and left when he was 14. She was heaven sent and she loved Tyler deeply. Even though Mary dressed differently than most people we knew, Tyler was always proud of her friendship. Every afternoon, she walked to his school and sat on a bench in the hallway until he found her.

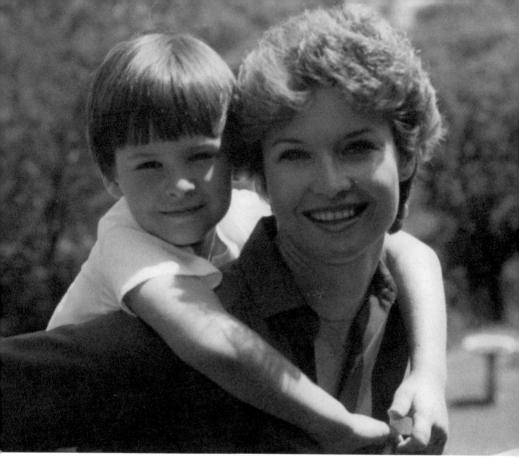

In Texas, I lived only a few minutes from the television station so I spent a lot of valuable time with Tyler.

The bond between Tyler and Mary was proved when I took her to have her eyes checked. She was nervous and was dwarfed by the huge examination chair. Tyler must have sensed her uneasiness and slipped into the chair with Mary when the lights went out. I was shocked that she did so well in responding to letters the doctor was flashing on the wall, until I heard Tyler whispering the answers to her.

Thank God that mothering is not reserved only for mothers. Tyler and I were so fortunate that Mary came into our lives and nurtured him during important years of his development. Several years later, my story of Mary appeared in *Chicken Soup for the Mother's Soul.*

By 1984, I was comfortable in my position at KXAS. The American Women in Radio and Television named me the top television newscaster in the Dallas-Fort Worth market. It was a wonderful honor because I was the first woman to receive the award.

Even with my success in Texas, my Oklahoma roots were calling. Balancing my personal life was a huge priority for me. I was tired of working nights because of the toll it was taking on my family. As women entered the work force and blazed trails to the top, the role of mother was not easily accommodated. I was the only mother in the newsroom in Oklahoma City and Dallas-Fort Worth. It was a balancing act that tore at my heart strings. If Tyler was sick, I was at work or I called in sick. Demanding careers and successful mothering, especially if you are a single parent, are an extremely challenging road.

Every spring on the anniversary of the time I signed my contract with KXAS, I received a call from KTVY general manager Lee Allan Smith, inquiring if I was ready to come home. Lee Allan's call in the spring of 1984 struck a chord. It was an excruciating decision. It was not about money, but it was one of those pivotal life moments—two paths were in front of me. One was an incredible career—top ten television market prime time news—and I loved it. But there was more to my life than my career—there was Tyler and family and Church of the Servant and Oklahoma.

In a newspaper article by Rhonda Glenn, a former television reporter, I was given much credit for the increased ratings at KXAS. She wrote, "Underneath all that womanly grace, there is a gritty female who outlasted five anchormen and has a lot to do with turning a devastated news operation into an award winner."

Rhonda knew how hard it was for me to leave that job—people just do not leave that kind of job. They are transferred, or they are fired, but they do not just quit. The salaries are too high and the perks of being a celebrity too ego-satisfying. To a broadcaster, a job in a top ten market, like a network job, means being king or queen of the media mountain.

Even though many perceived a move from a large market such as Dallas-Forth Worth to Oklahoma City as a step backward, for me it was a step toward lifelong friends and home.

SCOTT PELLEY

~ ~ ~ *"For news to have meaning, it has to have heart. Jane was the anchorwoman who, with her great and generous heart, gave purpose to our broadcasts at KXAS. I was her producer—and no producer ever had an easier time. With her sharp writing and sheer grace on the air, Jane was instantly a star. Demanding viewers were won over by her credibility—everyone else just simply loved to watch. My journey through journalism has taken me through many stages, but I have never met anyone who slipped so easily into the anchor chair. Many have followed Jane—but none have been her equal."*

VINCE ORZA

~ ~ ~ *{When I was a senior in high school in Shrub Oak, New York, Oklahoma City University sent a recruiter to my campus. The only thing I remember about the conversation was that Miss America was attending OCU. Any doubt that I had about attending OCU disappeared at that moment. Everything you have heard about Jane is true. She is warm, friendly, always pleasant, intelligent, articulate, thoughtful, professional, and of course, beautiful. We worked together at KOCO-TV and forged a lifetime friendship. When I was named the dean of the Meinders School of Business at OCU, Jane was the first to call with her congratulations. Who would have thought that Miss America would ever call me!"*

RON STAHL

~ ~ ~ *"Jane was one of the first people I met when I came to Oklahoma. We worked together at Channel 5 and at the Department of Tourism and Recreation. She is a rare person who is absolutely as nice as she seems. She wears the mantle of fame well and without pretension. She has a heart as big as the western Oklahoma sky, without the matching ego. In all of her roles, Jane was quietly, with dignity and grace, served as an outstanding ambassador for Oklahoma."*

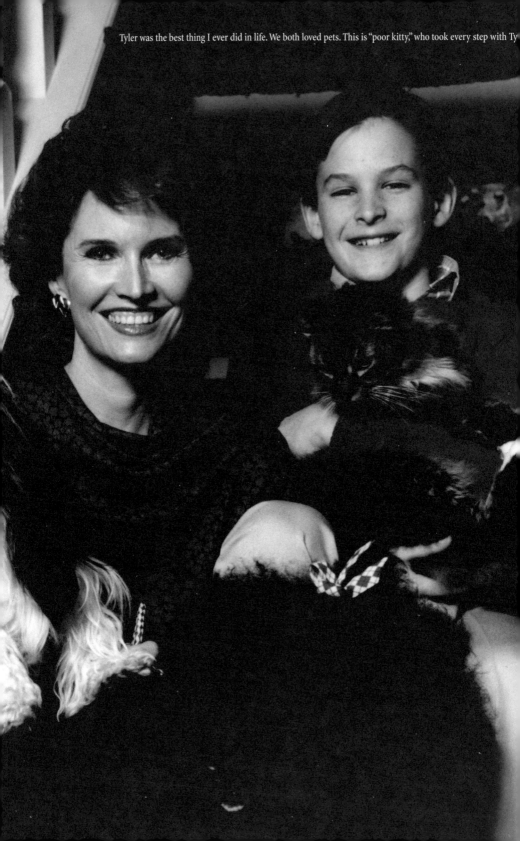

Tyler was the best thing I ever did in life. We both loved pets. This is "poor kitty," who took every step with Ty

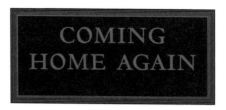

17

COMING HOME AGAIN

$\mathscr{B}$efore I began my new job in Oklahoma City, I did something that I had intended to do for a long time—spend more time with Tyler. I left Texas in the spring and took the summer off. I taught vacation Bible school at church and spent a lot of time with my family in Laverne. It was a summer that my little boy will never forget. It was a gift to me as well.

The great thing about my assignment at Channel 4 in Oklahoma City was that I was co-anchor of only the 5:00 p.m. and 6:00 p.m. news with Jerry Adams and Linda Cavanaugh. I was also a regular contributor to the 10:00 p.m. newscast, but my pieces were taped hours before. Unlike in my previous two jobs when I arrived home at 11:00 p.m., I was now free to be with Tyler by 7:00 p.m. and participate in many of his school activities I had been missing.

Lee Allan Smith was my mentor at Channel 4 who had taken a risk by hiring me as community relations director nearly 20 years before. He was so kind in negotiating my contract with the recognition that I was asking for special favors in not doing the 10:00 p.m. newscast. At many stations, news bosses insisted that the same anchors appear on all major evening newscasts.

Wayne moved back to Oklahoma before I did. Things were not working out as we planned, so we soon parted company. As a writer, he had given me great encouragement to begin preserving the memories of my life. Fortunately, I did begin chronicling my experiences, no doubt a preliminary exercise for this memoir.

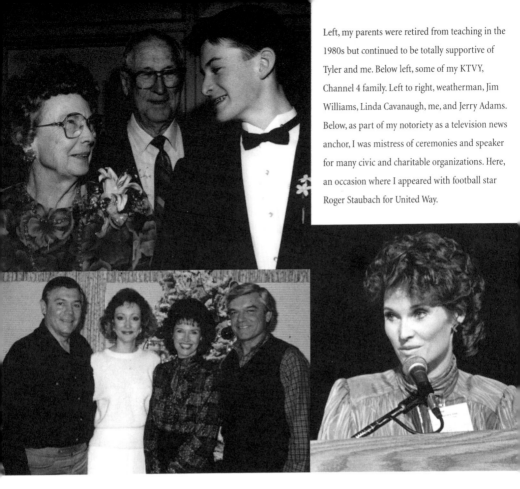

Left, my parents were retired from teaching in the 1980s but continued to be totally supportive of Tyler and me. Below left, some of my KTVY, Channel 4 family. Left to right, weatherman, Jim Williams, Linda Cavanaugh, me, and Jerry Adams. Below, as part of my notoriety as a television news anchor, I was mistress of ceremonies and speaker for many civic and charitable organizations. Here, an occasion where I appeared with football star Roger Staubach for United Way.

Tyler and I were so happy to be back among friends in Oklahoma. I quickly reestablished friendships and contacts with newsmakers and elected officials. I went on the air at Channel 4 on September 10, 1984. Linda Cavanaugh and I were probably the first female news team in America. We became fast friends, sharing not only a passion for broadcast journalism, but a dedication to family. Linda is a brilliant journalist and a really fun person. I love her, as well as her family.

Because Tyler was a little older and was in school all day, I had more time to be involved in community affairs. I joined worthy organizations and was selected for Leadership Oklahoma City and for the first board of Leadership Oklahoma, excellent groups that worked toward improving skills for future community leaders.

Preparing for just one major newscast block each day was a pleasant experience, even when we went on the road. In November, 1986, KTVY general manager Bob Finke decided that we should leave the studio and broadcast evening newscasts from six towns around the state. We broadcast live from Duncan, Purcell, Shawnee, El Reno, Enid, and Woodward, all in one week. It was a major technological achievement because a 35-person crew went ahead of us, making certain all the microphones and electrical hookups worked. The road crew operated from a 40-foot remote production truck.

My career path seems to be a journey of peaks and valleys and I was certainly responsible for some of the valleys. Because of my deep trust in Lee Allan Smith, I had not worried about renegotiating my contract at Channel 4 during the summer of 1987. As my contract ran out, Lee Allan was replaced as general manager when the station was sold. New management came in and made several bottom line decisions that changed the entire Oklahoma City television market. They offered me the early morning schedule at a greatly reduced salary. The reality of television news is that top salaries go to late night news anchors.

If I wanted to maintain the current lifestyle that Tyler and I enjoyed, including a lovely home with a big mortgage, I was going to have to return to the 10:00 news. Tyler and I made the decision. In July, 1987, I accepted an offer from KOCO-TV for the 6:00 p.m. and 10:00 p.m. newscasts.

It was big news—television anchors in Oklahoma City were playing musical chairs. Jerry Adams and I both were leaving Channel 4 for Channel 5—so were Butch and Ben McCain, entertainers with a popular morning show. Jack Bowen left Channel 5 for Channel 9, replacing Roger Cooper who went to weekend news shows. Gerry Harris, who had co-anchored with Jack Bowen, was given the noon and 5:00 p.m. anchor job at Channel 5.

One of my neatest assignments at Channel 5 was to salute Oklahoma schools and instructors in features pieces that aired on the prime time evening newscasts. I interviewed innovative and dedicated teachers and school administrators who were joining the television station's effort to address literacy and education issues. It was called Project Challenge. As a part of the emphasis on lifelong learning, I enrolled in a Ph.D. program at OU and received nine hours of graduate work in communications.

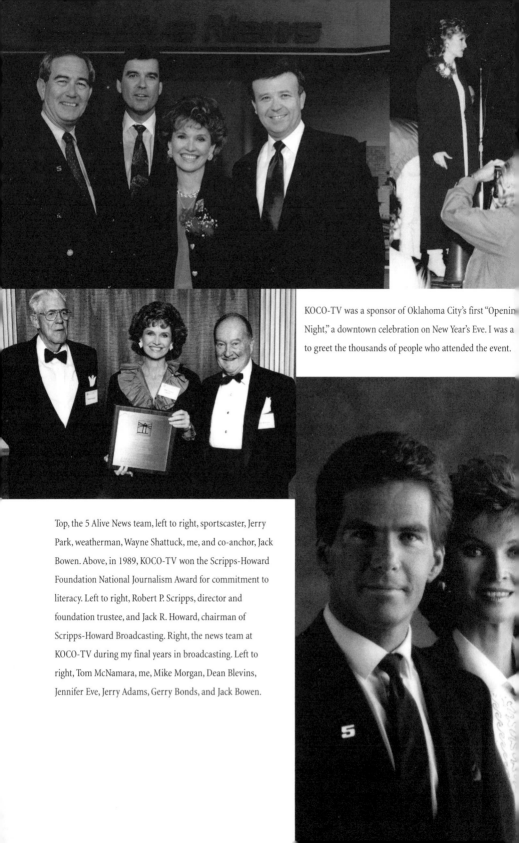

KOCO-TV was a sponsor of Oklahoma City's first "Openin[g] Night," a downtown celebration on New Year's Eve. I was a[ble] to greet the thousands of people who attended the event.

Top, the 5 Alive News team, left to right, sportscaster, Jerry Park, weatherman, Wayne Shattuck, me, and co-anchor, Jack Bowen. Above, in 1989, KOCO-TV won the Scripps-Howard Foundation National Journalism Award for commitment to literacy. Left to right, Robert P. Scripps, director and foundation trustee, and Jack R. Howard, chairman of Scripps-Howard Broadcasting. Right, the news team at KOCO-TV during my final years in broadcasting. Left to right, Tom McNamara, me, Mike Morgan, Dean Blevins, Jennifer Eve, Jerry Adams, Gerry Bonds, and Jack Bowen.

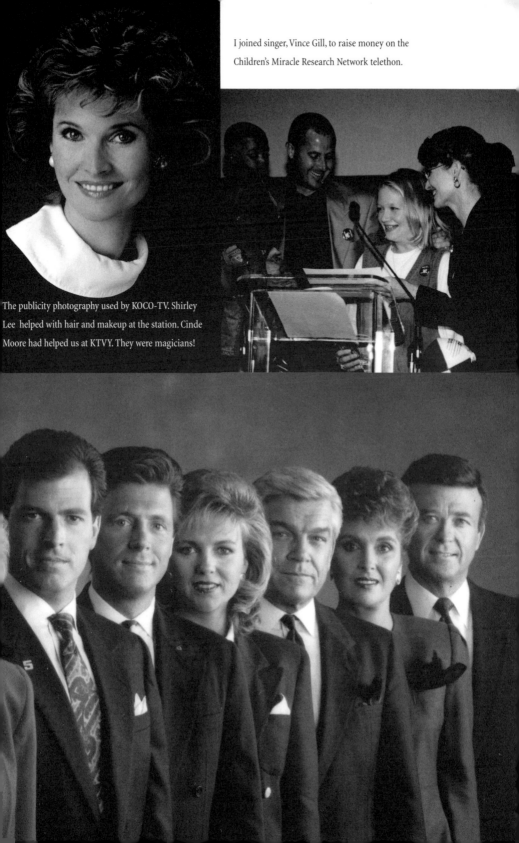

I joined singer, Vince Gill, to raise money on the Children's Miracle Research Network telethon.

The publicity photography used by KOCO-TV. Shirley Lee helped with hair and makeup at the station. Cinde Moore had helped us at KTVY. They were magicians!

I also was allowed to talk about family education issues in a special series on Channel 5 that featured Oklahoma families appearing live through video conferencing facilities at the state's vocational technical schools. I learned much about how normal people viewed their government's role in providing a quality education for their children.

In July, 1989, I was asked to appear with many other Oklahomans at the opening ceremonies of the United States Olympic Festival in Memorial Stadium in Norman. I joined a cast with stars such as Mickey Mantle, James Garner, Bob Hope, Jimmy Webb, Patti Page, Roger Miller, Abe Lemons, Bobby Murcer, Steve Owens, Allie Reynolds, Jim Shoulders, and Barry Switzer to celebrate the beginning of the Olympic Festival, an incredible ceremony that was produced largely through the efforts of Lee Allan Smith.

In September, 1989, the University of Oklahoma football team was in trouble when its top quarterback candidate was sent to prison on drug charges. OU was looking for a quarterback, and sports writer John Rohde, in *The Daily Oklahoman,* suggested that I be considered along with other anchorwomen and sportscasters such as Al Eschbach and Dean Blevins. Rohde wrote, "Just about anybody would suffice...It's simple. Just get the ball from center, turn around, and give it to somebody. If you see a hole, run through it." John must not have known that my sport was basketball, not football.

In 1990, Jack Bowen, who had begun with me at KOCO-TV 16 years before, returned from three years at Channel 9. Tom McNamara co-anchored the 6:00 p.m. and 10:00 p.m. shows with me, along with weatherman Mike Morgan, and sportscaster Dean Blevins. Myron Patton anchored the noon news and Jerry Adams, Chad Myers, and Jerry Park did weekend duty. Gerry Bonds, Butch and Ben McCain, and Jennifer Eve were also under contract.

At Channel 5 I continued to be active in civic organizations. My interest in education provided many opportunities to serve the community. Church of the Servant remained at the center of my life outside of work, whether it was as a member of the choir, helping women's ministries, or serving on the Administrative Council.

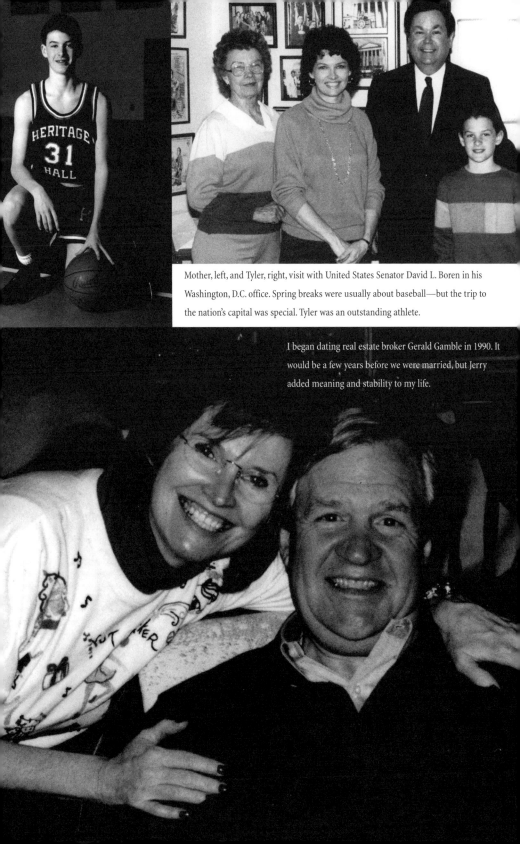

Mother, left, and Tyler, right, visit with United States Senator David L. Boren in his Washington, D.C. office. Spring breaks were usually about baseball—but the trip to the nation's capital was special. Tyler was an outstanding athlete.

I began dating real estate broker Gerald Gamble in 1990. It would be a few years before we were married, but Jerry added meaning and stability to my life.

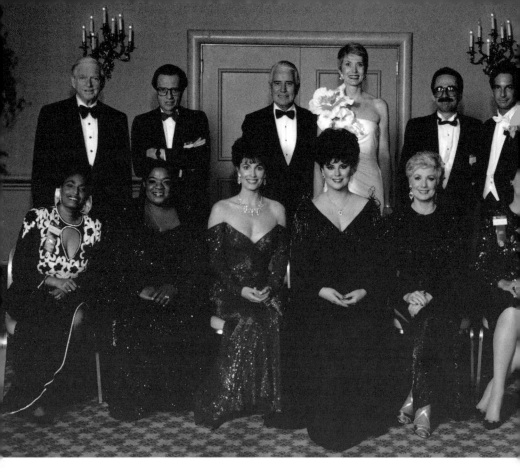

Governor Henry Bellmon appointed me to chair the "Oklahoma Reunion," an innovative program to involve Oklahomans in getting back to their roots in cities and towns where they were born or grew up. That government position followed my appointment by Governor George Nigh to the Oklahoma Commission on the Status of Women.

Several things happened in the early 1990s to cause me to seriously consider retiring from television. I had spent much of my son's life never being home at night and I saw his days at home numbered. I wanted to be with him more before he left home for college.

I also was approaching my mid-forties, a time when so many of the self-defining parts of my life were slipping away. It was a bit of a mid-life crisis. There was no doubt that my job was vulnerable because we were not number one in the market. I was more expensive and older than other women anchors. And, I was ready to leave.

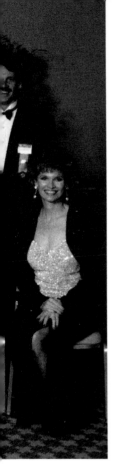

I was one of the judges for the 1990 Miss America Pageant that chose the 10 finalists. I was incredibly impressed with the new group of state winners. How smart and talented the girls were! My fellow judges, front to row, left to right, *New York Post* columnist Florence Anthony, actresses Nell Carter, Cynthia Sikes, Delta Burke, and Shirley Jones, opera star Gianna D'Angelo, and me. Standing, writer Sidney Sheldon, television talk show host Larry King, actor John Forsythe, motivational speaker Jeanne Swanner Robertson, film executive Jerry Rife, choreographer and director Thommie Walsh, and television host Ray Murray.

The surprise of aging brought all of that to a level of awareness. The physical changes were fully upon me. My arms were not long enough for me to read the newspaper. Almost overnight, my vision changed. I noticed I was saying "what?" more often and it was not just my mumbling teenage son. Instead of being bloated just once a month, my waistline seemed to be expanded most of the time, and it was best to avoid looking at my face in a magnifying glass for the new lines and sags I would see. To complete a good paragraph including any historical data required a committee of my best friends.

It was all a surprise, this getting older. For some reason, I just never thought it would happen to me—certainly not so quickly. I was so busy in my younger years that I never thought about middle age and growing even older.

In 1992, I had to look to the future when my parents would be gone, my son might live far away in his own life, and I might be living alone. I was over 40 and still single. I had to face the fact that I was in an industry that thrived on youthfulness. My looks that had always dictated my career and self image were becoming diminished.

I was not distraught about aging, but I wanted to find a way to reconcile the feelings of loss and fears about the future. I wanted a way to be hopeful about the rest of my life. I did not want to be startled by the next season of life—I wanted to prepare for it, physically, emotionally, financially, and most importantly, spiritually.

As a Christian, I had a real ebb and flow kind of relationship with God. I always went to the church and worshipped Him. I prayed, but often would fall asleep or get distracted by my endless "to do" list. God and I were really close, especially when I had an emergency. But it was apparent that I did not have the kind of bedrock relationship with God that some other people seemed to build upon.

I did not know God's character enough to completely trust Him. I did not know the Bible well enough to be obedient. Looking ahead into my next phase of life, I was saddened by the inevitable losses, fearful about being alone, concerned about financial issues, and unsure about my spiritual state.

After 17 years in television news, I believed I needed a career change, but I also needed an identity review and a focus for the future. I determined in my soul to reach for a deeper relationship with God. Little did I know His plans for a new career and a blessed marriage.

In the late spring of 1992, I made a decision to retire from Channel 5 and become the full-time spokesperson for the 25 federal, state, and private institutions that make up the Oklahoma Health Center. In addition, I would serve as vice president of the Presbyterian Health Foundation.

I had no problem making the career change. My days in television were over—but my future of giving back to Oklahoma was just beginning.

LINDA CAVANAUGH

~ ~ ~ *"Jane and I met when she came to Channel 4 as an anchor. It did not take long to find a common bond—dedication to our children. Jane made career decisions based on the needs of her son, Tyler. I admired that. She put her responsibilities as a mother first—and that can be an unusual thing in the world of television. It is not surprising that Jane was among the first successful females in broadcasting. She has never been one to hide from challenges. Whether it was stepping out of a small town onto the world stage as Miss America or taking over the reins of the Oklahoma Department of Tourism with its multi-million dollar budget, Jane has succeeded in everything.*
She has the depth of character to make the right decision the first time. She has a sense of self that keeps everything in perspective. I have never known her to be blinded by the bright lights of "celebrity" or to veer from the path of what is important to her— family and faith. When people say that Oklahoma's greatest resource is her people, they must surely be talking about Oklahomans like Jane Jayroe."

TOM KIRBY

~ ~ ~ *"Jane tackled every kind of news assignment. Her time as Miss America and beyond had brought her into contact with almost every town in Oklahoma. It was nearly impossible to toss a news story at her for which she had no "contacts." She had met the mayor or she could describe the block where the event happened. She had devoted her life to Oklahoma and that showed up every time a director punched her camera on the air. You could see it in her eyes."*

BOBBIE ROE

~ ~ ~ *"Jane's high-profile public life would suggest that her identity has been shaped largely by her professional roles. But who Jane is springs first and foremost from her relationship with God. She daily listens for God's guidance in prayer, and she seeks counsel form friends and mentors of similar faith. Because she is open to receive inspiration from many sources, Jane often gets big ideas that develop into educational and spiritual opportunities for the Oklahoma community. She brings her ideas to fruition by engaging others' gifts, instead of trying to orchestrate events with sole attention to herself.*

While I have been privileged to share some of the fruits of Jane's big ideas, I will always cherish the small gifts of our friendship. We pray for each other's sons. We chat by e-mail whenever one of us needs to entrust a heart's burden to the other. And, although she claims not to cook, she even made me soup after I had minor surgery."

LEE ALLAN SMITH

~ ~ ~ *"Most Oklahomans know that one of the greatest moments in Jane's life was when she was crowned Miss America. However, I would like to think she believes one of her great moments was when she returned to her home state of Oklahoma from a very successful career as the number one anchorwoman in the Dallas/Fort Worth television market. She returned to Oklahoma City in 1974 to work for Channel 4. She is a great asset to Oklahoma, as she adds her charm, grace, and talent to the many community affairs in which she is involved."*

KAREN VINYARD WADDELL

~ ~ ~ *"Jane is more beautifully spiritually than she is physically,*
even though men and women describe her as "drop-dead
gorgeous." She has always reminded me of a more softened
Jacqueline Kennedy—beautiful natural freshness with an inner
spirit reflecting so elegantly outside. She has a spirit that reflects
kindness and goodness and love that it can only be
divinely inspired."

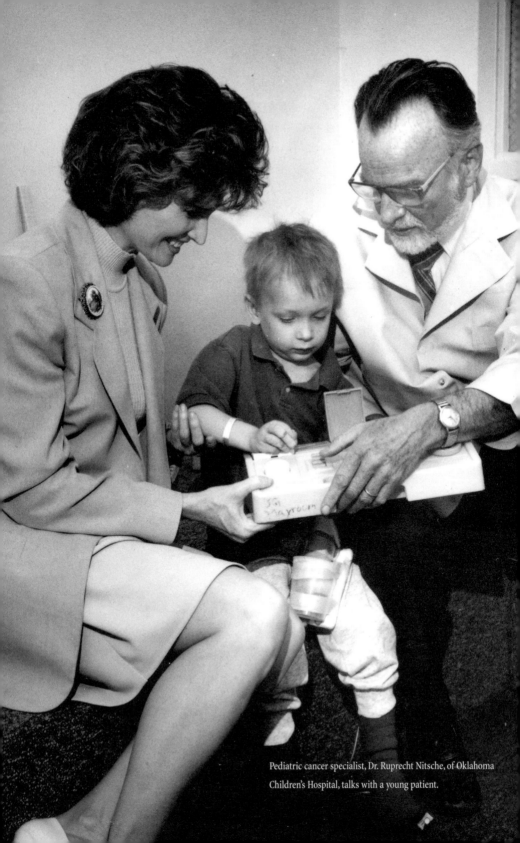

Pediatric cancer specialist, Dr. Ruprecht Nitsche, of Oklahoma Children's Hospital, talks with a young patient.

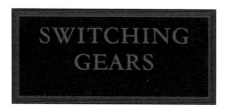

18

SWITCHING GEARS

One of the great things about producing and hosting television specials on projects that involved the Oklahoma Health Center (OHC) was my daily contact with Jean Gumerson, president of the Presbyterian Health Foundation (PHF). Jean was such a role model for women in charitable and civic causes. She selflessly led the way in helping me prepare programs for the media and promote the Oklahoma Health Center, an incredible resource for Oklahoma.

While at OHC, I also learned to appreciate the decades of service to Oklahoma by Stanton L. Young. It was his vision and leadership that has made all the difference in that complex. When I had an idea that could further the success of OHC, Stanton was available, with mountains of information on who to contact and how to proceed.

My goal at OHC was to bridge the gap between the accomplishments of the many facets of OHC and the public's need to know and understand more about health care and the fight against disease. My friend, Karen Waddell, had helped me created the proposal for OHC even though it could cost her agency future business. She was such a generous friend.

In April, 1993, I inaugurated "Jane Jayroe's Medical Journal," a 30-minute television program, the first in a series of programs to air on Oklahoma television stations. The first segment of the initial program revealed plans for a new Oklahoma City clinic for children with cancer. The Jimmy Everest Center for Cancer was named for 17-year-old Jimmy Everest who lost his life to cancer. On the television show was a heart wrenching discussion with Jim and Christy Everest about their son's battle with cancer and their willingness to turn tragedy into hope through raising funds for a new facility.

Also on the initial program was an AIDS research story that highlighted the international attention being received by Dr. Jordan Tang of the Oklahoma Medical Research Foundation. Dr. Tang and his staff had created a new gene which might be used in gene therapy in the fight against AIDS.

A final segment included an interview with Dr. Warren "Sonny" Jackman from the University of Oklahoma Health Sciences Center. Dr. Jackman talked about a relatively minor heart procedure that was life-changing for patients. The procedure, called radiofrequency catheter ablation, works by nonsurgically destroying a small area of the heart in which electrical malfunctions are occurring, causing episodes of rapid heartbeat. Dr. Jackman was a pioneer and patients from around the world came to Oklahoma City to be under his care.

I learned so much about fighting disease and I was privileged to meet so many men and women who spent their every waking hour looking for cures for the diseases and conditions that affect so many people in the world.

The series of programs on every imaginable health topic, including breast cancer research, sports medicine, aging, heart disease, and arthritis, was sponsored by Macklanburg-Duncan Company and Boatmen's Bank, and was produced by the Presbyterian Health Foundation and Karim E. Karim Productions. I also provided health reports on KOCO-TV on the 5:00 p.m. news and on "Good Morning Oklahoma."

In addition to developing and hosting "Jane Jayroe's Medical Journal," I appeared at dozens of medical forums with leading physicians and researchers. I discovered that Oklahomans really wanted to know the latest about diseases that were affecting their lives.

It was so rewarding to have an opportunity as part of my career to be an active volunteer in the community. I was an active board member of The Oklahoma Health Center Foundation, and the OU Breast Health Institute with two of my favorite people, Dr. Debra Mitchell and Dr. Allen Hollingsworth. My friend, Patricia Browne, recruited me for that involvement as well as kept me involved in Children's Medical Research. It was a joy to work with the American Red Cross as part of my job. Dee Jackson was the person who had helped me create the "Volunteer Connection," a program to recruit people to volunteer in the community. Dee was an angel. As always, I remained active at Church of the Servant and Oklahoma City University.

I had the opportunity for a few years to serve as a trustee on the Sarkeys Foundation in Norman. That was such a gift to be able to help direct funds to worthwhile organizations.

Greater than the fulfilling community activity that went along with this new job experience was the joy of being a parent with normal working hours. Tyler was an easy child to raise, but he did not have an easy time

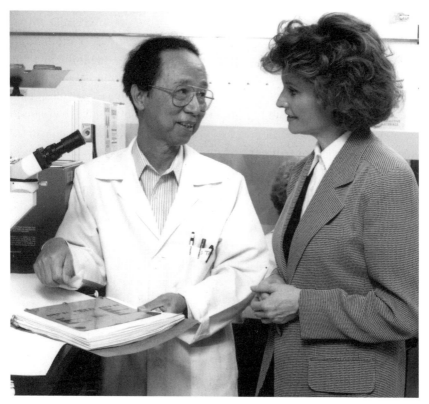

Dr. Jordan Tang of the Oklahoma Medical Research Foundation appeared on the television program, "Jane Jayroe's Medical Journal."

growing up. He wrote in an essay once that "growing up without a father was difficult, but it was more difficult to grow up with a mother who was a celebrity in a state that had so few." It was fun for him when he was little to have some of the special attention of my career like meeting his sports heroes—but that faded into self consciousness as he grew older.

He attended Quail Creek Elementary in the OKC school system where he had outstanding teachers. I transferred him to a private school after that, rather than send him to a fifth-year center. With my public education background, I was reluctant to send him to a private school, but the size of the public school and the concept of a huge building with one grade just did not seem like a good option to me. Because Tyler was gifted academically and loved sports, I wanted him to have some of the advantages that I had growing up in a small school and being able to participate in a variety of activities. He received that at Heritage Hall.

Tyler will say his experience at Heritage Hall was far from perfect, but he made the best of it. He was an outstanding student, a national merit finalist, and a gifted member of the golf and basketball teams. Tyler never gave me a moment's trouble, but I hurt for the problems my mistakes had caused him. He would say that it all served him well in the long run. But all parents know that there is nothing more painful than watching your child struggle, especially when you feel responsible for causing the struggle.

It was difficult to be a single parent with a demanding career. Tyler made it as easy as possible. My extended family played an incredible role. From the beginning, Tyler belonged as much to my parents as to me. He loved going to Laverne. The security of my parents and that little town that changed so little were much of the base that allowed Tyler to become such a mature and stable young man. My sister and her three sons were also very much our family as well as her new husband, Frank Elmore.

An enormous blessing that occurred during my life after television was my marriage to Jerry Gamble. Our wedding was on April 9, 1994, at the little chapel at Church of the Servant. Tyler was a senior in high school but Jerry had been a part of our lives for many years. Jerry and I had so much in common. He grew up in a small town in east Texas and, like me, had participated in every possible activity. He came from a wonderful family where his mother became a school teacher after her three children were in school.

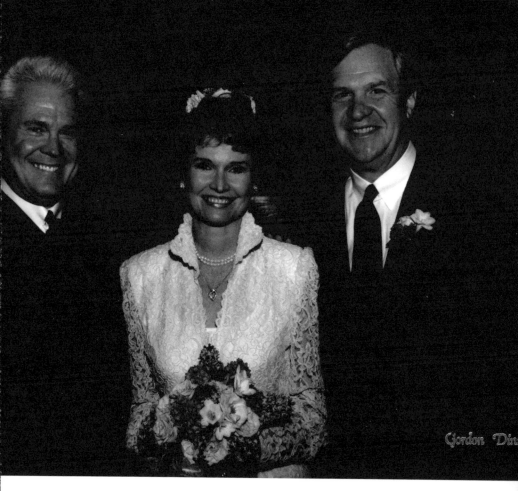

Jerry and I were married by Dr. Norman Neaves on April 9, 1994.

Jerry grew up in the Methodist Church, and in fact, my pastor, Norman Neaves, had introduced us months before we ever dated. I can remember a time many years before I met Jerry that I was visiting with Norman and telling him how much I needed to change and be a person who was more assertive and practical. Norman told me that he would wish for me that I marry someone who would be the kind of balance for me that would allow me to be more fully the person that I was created to be, rather than trying to be someone else. In other words, while it is important for me to be responsible, which I am, my gifts flow from the person that God created me to be—emotional, artistic, and creative. When I try to flatten that out, and make it hardened, it is not very successful.

Jerry has given me many gifts, but the greatest gift is just as Norman described so many years ago. Because Jerry by his nature is very mature, practical, and stable, it has allowed me such greater freedom and comfort to be who God has called me to be. I believe I have softened Jerry's heart a little in the process as well.

I am so proud to be Mrs. Gerald Gamble. Jerry, without any outside help, went to the University of Oklahoma and was named "outstanding man" his senior year. He was awarded a Woodrow Wilson Fellowship and received his masters degree from Stanford University. He returned to Oklahoma where he worked for his uncle, Harold Brand, and went to night school at OCU where he obtained his juris doctor degree, graduating number one in his class. Jerry has had a very successful career as a commercial and industrial real estate broker in Oklahoma City with his own company, Gerald L. Gamble Company. Did I mention that he has enormous energy?

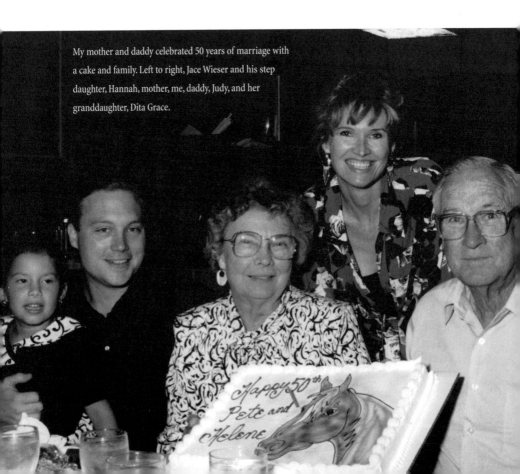

My mother and daddy celebrated 50 years of marriage with a cake and family. Left to right, Jace Wieser and his step daughter, Hannah, mother, me, daddy, Judy, and her granddaughter, Dita Grace.

He is a fun and energetic person to live with. He is a workaholic, but I do not mind that. He is not subtle in his opinions, which I have learned to live with. Jerry has been a very important community leader in Oklahoma City. For the first time in my life, I was a "civic spouse," which was great fun. Jerry was elected chairman of the Oklahoma City Chamber of Commerce in 1997, another in a long line of organizations that he headed in Oklahoma City. I am very proud of Jerry's great mind, passionate heart for service, and loyalty. He has been very helpful to Tyler. We have a blessed life and share a love of church, OCU, travel, pets, and music.

One of the bonuses of marrying Jerry was getting a new set of friends and family. Jerry's mother, Eloise, lives in Jefferson, Texas. His sister, Anne, is married to Duard Pyle and has two grown children, Julie and Philip, who is married to Bea and has Emily. Jerry's brother, Jim, and Marty Newby Gamble have two grown daughters, Wendy and Misty. Marty was a special joy for me. Even though she has lived in Los Angeles for many years, Marty grew up in Alva and her father was the football coach at Northwestern State

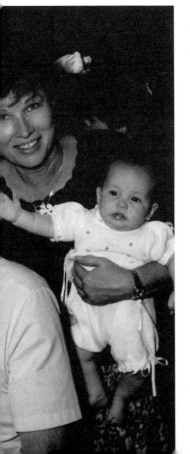

University. Marty was an Alpha Chi Omega at OU and her birthday is almost the same day as mine. We have a rich friendship.

Patricia Browne, the wife of one of Jerry's best friends, Henry Browne, Jr., became one of my best friends. Initially, I was not really comfortable in a lot of Jerry's social environments. I had always been a working girl and did not know many Oklahoma City people outside of my career experience. Patricia welcomed me with open arms and we fell instantly into "like" with each other.

Patricia died very unexpectedly in the fall of 2000—a devastating blow for her family and friends. I wrote this in remembrance of her. I believe it captures Patricia, and teaches all of us a few lessons.

Patricia's Special Wisdom
Don't waste your life with worry or regrets.
Spend time wisely with people and projects that really matter.
Work and play out of a sense of love and joy, not duty.
Don't let dreary details take away an opportunity to be
        with someone you love.
Never take a day for granted.
And never pass up a good dessert.

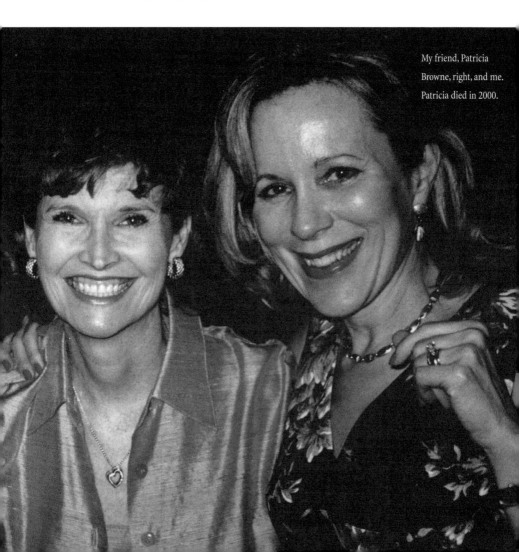

My friend, Patricia Browne, right, and me. Patricia died in 2000.

In 1994, I was asked to read a modern Christmas story for *The Daily Oklahoman*'s Christmas Access line which contained several holiday features to which callers could listen. Former Governor George Nigh read "The Night Before Christmas," Dr. Bobby Boyles read "One Solitary Life," cartoonist Jim Lange read "Yes, Virginia There is a Santa Claus," and I read "A Cup of Christmas Tea," by Tom Hegg.

My reading created a stir. Robert E. Lee, writing in *The Daily Oklahoman*, said, "This new addition may not yet be considered classical or traditional. But in my opinion, that's where it's headed." The story was about paying off credit cards, older folks suffering strokes, and other modern day problems. But it was also about love which is, after all, what Christmas is all about.

I continued to put my thoughts about my life's struggles on paper. I wanted to somehow share my battles, and ultimate victories by God's grace, with a wider audience than just my friends and an occasional audience.

One project to help people was the release in February, 1995, of a tape series of inspirational messages by six Oklahoma City ministers and lay leaders.

I worked with senior ministers, Don Alexander, Michael Anderson, and Gene Garrison, and my own pastor, Norman Neaves, to provide words of comfort and advice to people who juggled many roles and needed just a few minutes of peace to reflect on how to make our lives better, or to just be inspired for the day. Also providing taped messages were Robert Henry, former attorney general and dean of the OCU School of Law, and C. Stephen Lynn, chief executive officer of Sonic Industries, Inc. We raised some money for Childrens Medical Research and hopefully inspired some folks as well.

An unusual writing project for me was a weight loss article published by *McCalls* magazine in March, 1996. The magazine's cover hyped the story, "Drop 20 pounds—Miss America's weight-loss plan."

In the article, titled "Miss America Shapes Up," I talked about how extra weight had crept up on me in middle age, how I became an expert at covering up. After all, I was too busy enjoying life to worry about weight gain. The magazine included a photograph of me up 22 pounds from my beauty pageant weight. I tried to emphasize a combination of correct eating habits and exercise that helped me take off the unwanted pounds.

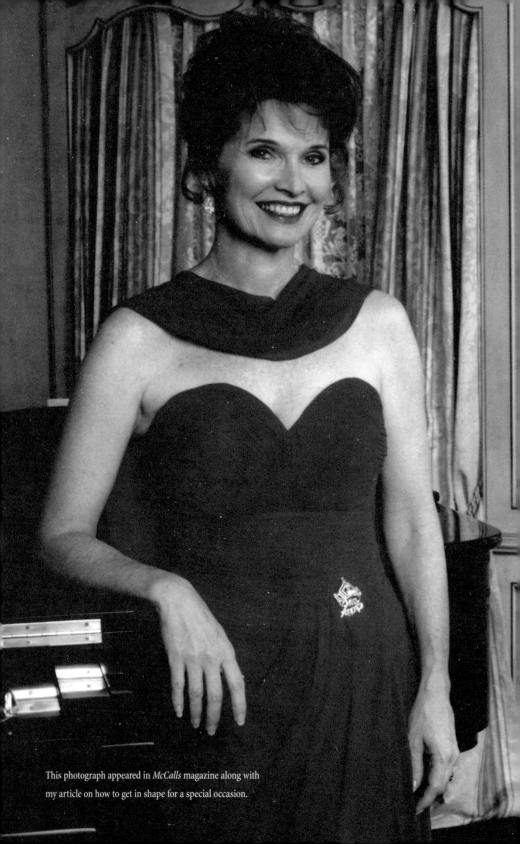

This photograph appeared in *McCalls* magazine along with
my article on how to get in shape for a special occasion.

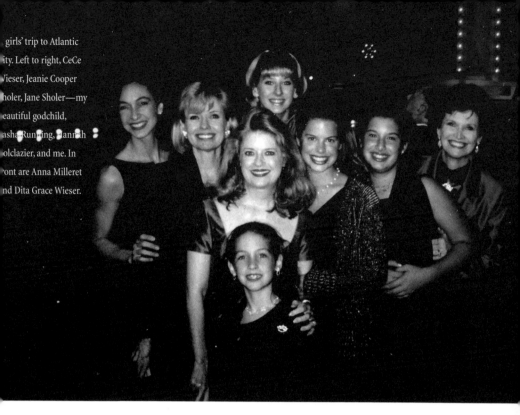

As much as I wanted to lose weight, 15 pounds, I really wanted to be published in a national magazine. I had wanted to write professionally for years, other than writing television news, and this was my chance.

In September, 1996, I was humbled by my selection as the first woman elected chair of the Oklahoma Academy for State Goals, a statewide public policy think tank. This organization had been a favorite activity of mine since I attended its first conference with Governor Bellmon and Doug Fox in 1985. This was a deeper interest in Oklahoma than I had experienced in any other environment. The annual conferences, the non-partisan nature, and the statewide focus made the Oklahoma Academy a worthwhile volunteer activity.

Former chair Burns Hargis convinced me to accept the position as the first woman to chair the academy. Director Julie Conatser made me look good—she makes every chair look good. I worked alongside other academy officers Rodger Randle, Dave Lopez, Martin Garber, and Howard Barnett. The Academy is where I got to know some of my favorite Oklahomans— H.E. "Gene" Rainbolt, Roger Webb, Ken Fergeson, Ron Howell, Bill

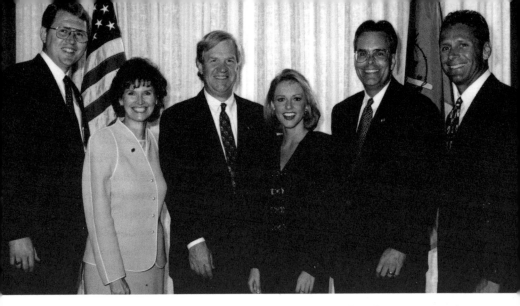

I was challenged by my work with the Oklahoma Academy for State Goals. Left to right, Congressman Frank Lucas, me, Jerry, Shawntel Smith Wuerch, Ron Howell, and Congressman Steve Largent.

McKamey, Mike Turpen, Lex Holmes, Mike Lapolla, Larkin Warner, Frederick Drummond, Clyde Wheeler, Bob McCormick, Jim Tolbert, and so many others. The best thing I did for the Academy was to recruit Cliff Hudson, chief executive officer of Sonic. He has left a lasting legacy on the organization.

In November of that year, I was asked to co-host "Discover Oklahoma," a program boosting Oklahoma's tourist destinations produced by the Oklahoma Department of Tourism and Recreation. I reported on stories from throughout the state, showing state parks, museums, bed and breakfasts, and other spots of interest. I learned so much about my native state. It was perfect training for my next job.

HENRY BROWNE, JR.

~ ~ ~ *"Jane represents what every parent would want their daughter to be—an intelligent, attractive, loving, and productive woman. She is a deeply dedicated wife, mother, and family member—true to the ethical and spiritual values she learned from her parents. Because of Jane's sincerity, integrity, and strong character, she has many friends, supporters, and communities cheering for her."*

KEN FERGESON

~ ~ ~ *"Serving with Jane on the board of the Oklahoma Academy for State goals, I discovered that in addition to her cool manner and professionalism, she was a deep thinker. She is consistently engaged and involved in anything to which she agrees to commit and lend her name. Jane's dedication to make Oklahoma a better place to live has been an inspiration to me and has encouraged me to do more for the state and its people."*

JEAN GUMERSON

~ ~ ~ *"My friendship with Jane began with us both being involved in volunteerism, the champagne of life. She was always ready to pitch in and help in any worthy cause.*
Jane is not just beautiful, she is caring and generous to all of Oklahoma. She was the perfect daughter, the perfect student, and is a friend who is never critical and demanding, but always wanting to help."

BURNS HARGIS

~ ~ ~ *"I first Jane while I was in law school. I had never met a Miss America so I was very impressed. The irony was, if anything, Jane was more humble than me. Her looks had taken her to the top, but her consummate graciousness has been her trademark ever since. No matter how prominent her position as Miss America, news anchor in a major market, or head of a large state agency, she has remained that polite, humble gal from Laverne. There is not a haughty bone in her body. She is truly one of Oklahoma's greatest assets."*

LORI HANSEN LANE

~ ~ ~ *"Jane has been a sweet and steadfast friend. I remember her tears of empathy flowing for me during a difficult time. I was at a Bible study with Jane and three other friends who were gathered around to pray for me. As we prayed, I found my attention diverted to the steady drip of Jane's tears upon my hand. Mere drops to some—a fountain of compassion to me. I will never forget that moment.*

Jane is a woman who loves and serves the Lord and who is available to Him for service—when and where he calls. Just as Esther was called "a woman for a time such as this," so is Jane. She is a woman who serves her state, her community, her church, and her God, and is my friend in "a time such as this."

JACKIE JONES

~ ~ ~ *"I love watching Jane in public, as countless women approach her, and she treats each one as a dear friend. Her eyes sparkly, she is fully engaged in what they are saying, and her smile lights up their faces and their days. Those of us who are blessed with special friendships with her receive the same treatment, plus, she supports and encourages, and reminds us of the incredible blessings we enjoy, even on our dark days. She also shares fashion tips when asked!"*

H.E. "GENE" RAINBOLT

~ ~ ~ *"Jane is an insightful leader, a persistent pursuer of perfection, an articulate institutional voice, a dedicated mother, a loyal friend, and in every possible way an extraordinary person with an uncompromising value system."*

CATHY LEICHTER

~ ~ ~ *"Jane has been connected to so many lives, touched so many people, and left kindness where ever she has been. She truly is created for a time such as this."*

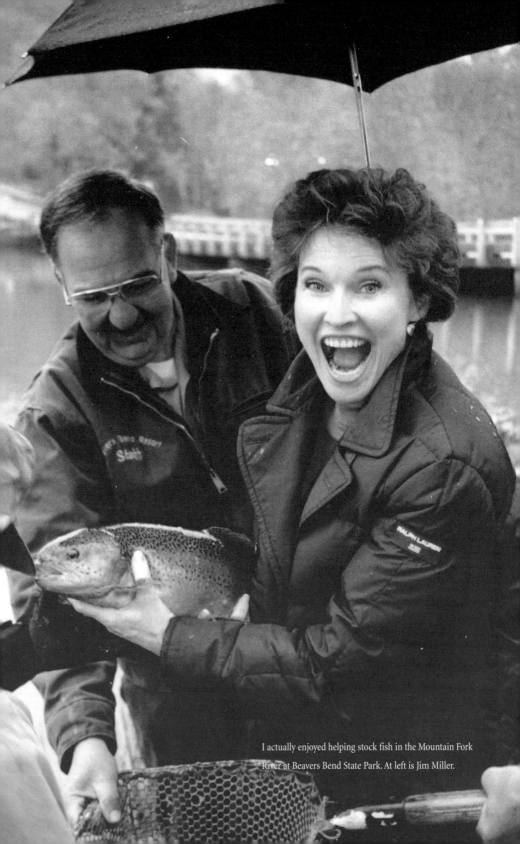

I actually enjoyed helping stock fish in the Mountain Fork River at Beavers Bend State Park. At left is Jim Miller.

19

BOOSTING TOURISM

*I*n February, 1999, Governor Frank Keating asked me to head the state's tourism efforts as Cabinet Secretary for Tourism and executive director of the Oklahoma Department of Tourism and Recreation. I was contacted initially by Kay Dudley, a woman I would grow to love. She was Governor Keating's director of appointments. Kay and the governor's chief of staff, Ken Lackey interviewed me. They must have believed I had enough of the qualities they were looking for, because my next interview was with the governor himself.

As usual, I had my detractors at the beginning. When I was appointed, Senator Dave Herbert of Midwest City told a reporter that I had a "name," but he questioned whether I had the administrative experience necessary to run a huge state agency. I accepted his concern as a challenge. As it turned out, Senator Herbert became one of my strongest allies in the State Senate. Lieutenant Governor Mary Fallin, chair of the State Tourism Commission, expressed confidence in me. She said, "Jane will make a great ambassador for the state of Oklahoma."

When Governor Keating asked me to take the tourism post, I knew it was God's call on my life and I did not hesitate to accept. When my friend, Sue Sewell, heard about my appointment, she called to congratulate me. She laughed and said, "You are fearless!" I laughed, too, because I was far from fearless but I was learning to be faithful to the call on my life.

It was tough duty from the beginning. On my third day on the job, I had to appear before a State Senate committee. I told the senators that

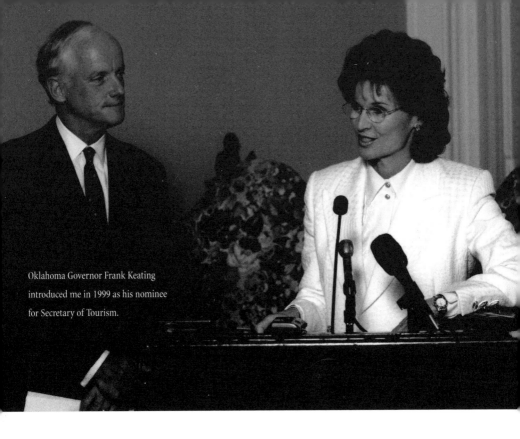

Oklahoma Governor Frank Keating introduced me in 1999 as his nominee for Secretary of Tourism.

Oklahoma must be sold, or promoted, as the greatest place to visit and live. I stepped into the crossfire between the governor and the legislature over the governor's proposal to sell some of the money-losing state lodges and most of the state-owned golf courses.

As the state's tourism director, I oversaw an annual budget of more than $60 million, with 1,300 employees, and the operation of 51 state parks, five state resorts, 11 golf courses, and a variety of marketing and development programs designed to enhance the economic impact of the state's tourism industry.

I was the first tourism director from a marketing and public relations background. I like to think that my training allowed me to energize the industry. I was on the road constantly, visiting our tourist locations and, more importantly, the great people who operated them. I went out of my way to make sure the state parks employees knew they were appreciated. I made so many new friends.

At Tourism, I depended greatly upon Leann Overstake, center, and Doug Enevoldsen, right, the deputy director of the agency. State Parks Director John Ressmeyer, at right in photo below, used his organizational talents to make great improvements in Oklahoma's state parks.

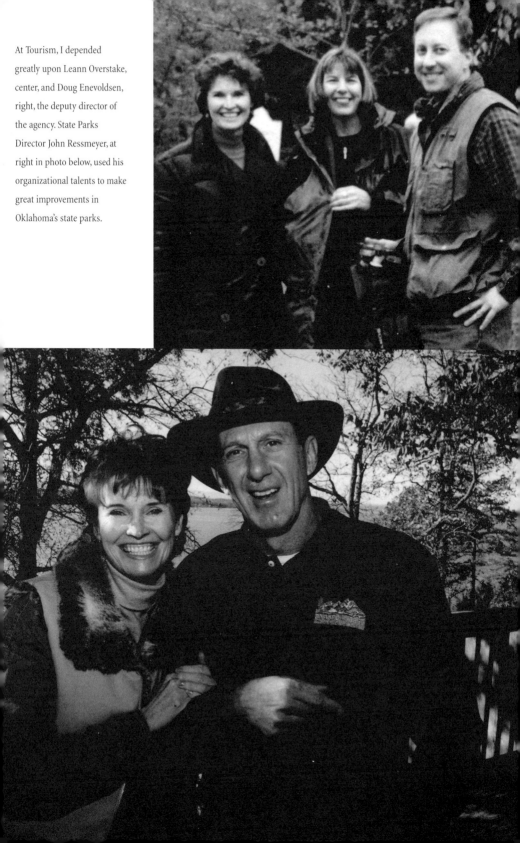

I was impressed with God's great creation that was contained in our state parks. When I visited beautiful Beavers Bend State Park near Broken Bow, I wrote in my journal: *The river, the lake, the trees, the wildlife, the smell of outdoor fires, the eagles, the hawks, the owls, the turkeys, the crisp air, the rainbow trout, the gold yeller trout, the rural people. This is exactly what I needed. The reminder of this privilege of affecting good people and places. Hopefully, its images to store in my heart.*

I appeared at many meetings of local chambers of commerce and civic clubs. I was completely confident of our department's direction and could stand and talk about tourism for hours. After one speech, I noted in my journal, "Look what God has done with me. Taking a girl who was so shy she almost would not get out of the car on the first day at a new school, and made her a speaker before thousands."

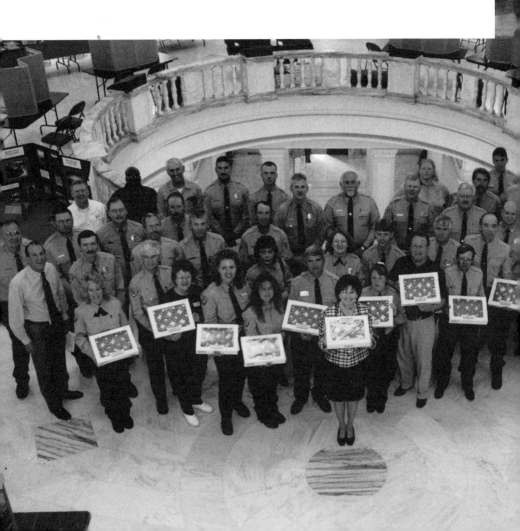

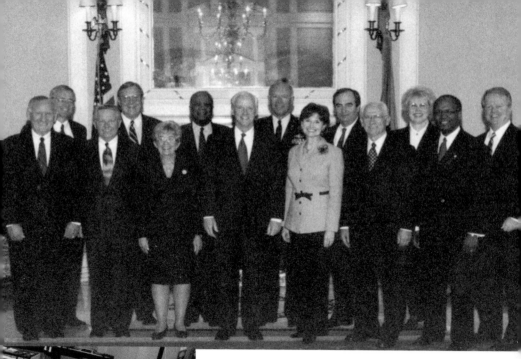

I was honored to be a member of Governor Frank Keating's cabinet. Left to right, front row, Brian Griffin, Norman Lamb, Bob Ricks, Kay Dudley, Governor Keating, me, Dr. Floyd Coppedge, Oscar Jackson, and Bob Sullivan. Back row, Howard Hendricks, Herschal Crow, Russell Perry, Harry Wyatt, III, Tom Daxon, and Pam Warren.

Left, the directors of Oklahoma's state parks pose with me in the rotunda of the State Capitol. With the help of tourism commissioner Hal Smith, we had Krispy Kreme donuts for legislators before they were available to the public in Oklahoma.

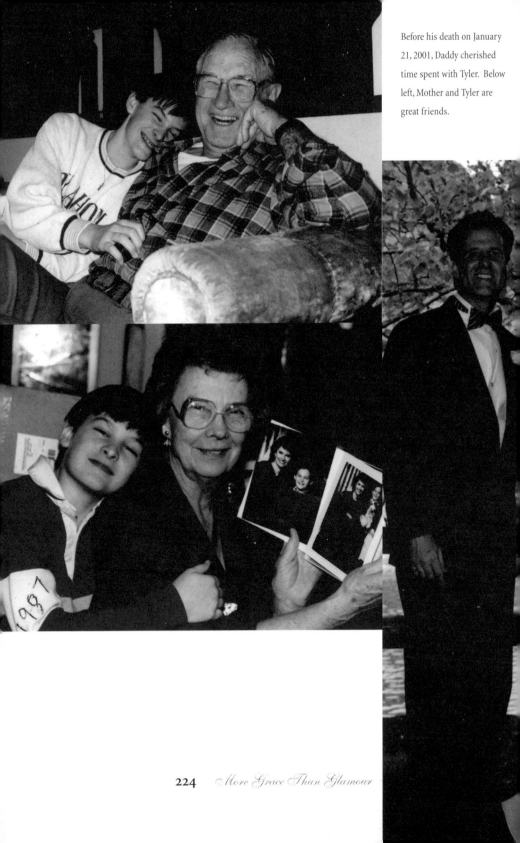

Before his death on January 21, 2001, Daddy cherished time spent with Tyler. Below left, Mother and Tyler are great friends.

Tyler married Elaine Gulotta on May 29, 1999. Left to right, Mike Gulotta, Madeline Gulotta, Elaine, Tyler, me, and Jerry.

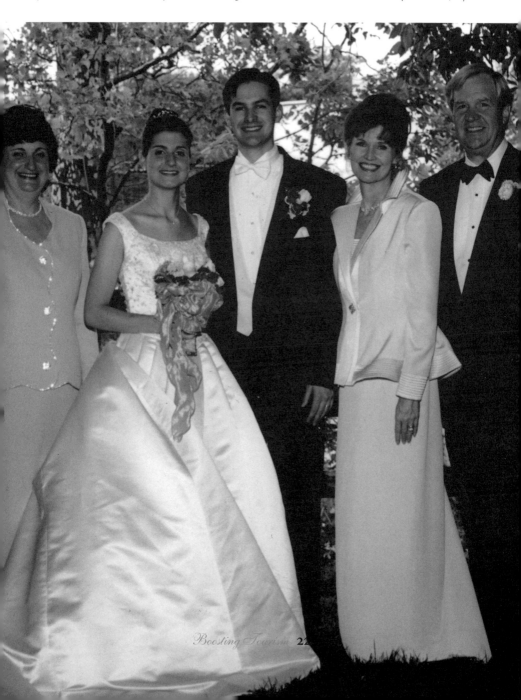

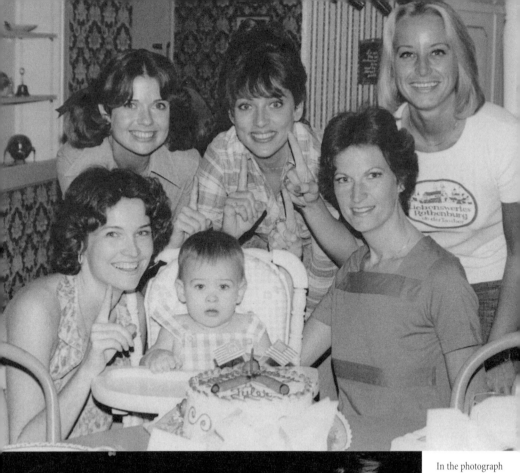

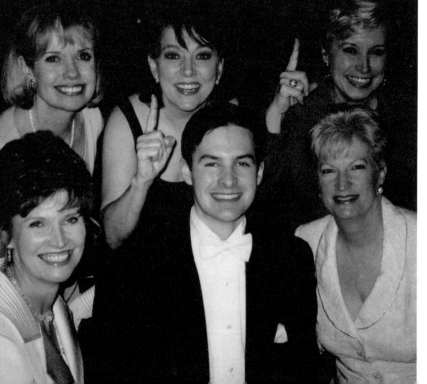

In the photograph above, my dear friends, top row, left to right, Jeanie Cooper, Kerry Robertson, and Vicki Kelley, and front row, Sue Wells, right, posed with me and baby Tyler on July 4, 1977, on his first birthday. In the photograph below, the same friends appeared with Tyler on his wedding day on May 29, 1999.

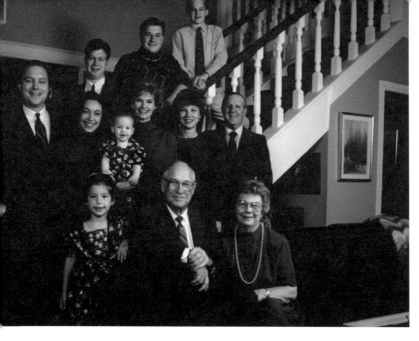

Our family had grown through the years. Back row, left to right, Jace Wieser, Dal Wieser, Cade Elmore, and Tyler. Middle row, Cece Wieser, holding Dita Grace, me, Judy Elmore, and Frank Elmore. In front, Hannah Colclazier, daddy, and mother.

Tyler was such a good student and great kid that I had promised him that if he made good grades in high school, I would try to send him to any college he wanted. I did not anticipate how upsetting it would be for me to see him leave Oklahoma. We visited some great universities throughout America and he was admitted to most of them, including Stanford University in California. He made the decision to attend Vanderbilt University in Nashville, Tennessee. It was the right choice for him and much easier on me. It was academically challenging, but also offered an environment in which he could grow socially. He fit in and made some of the most wonderful friends for life. He majored in history with a minor in Spanish and graduated magna cum laude and Phi Beta Kappa. In the summers, he interned for Governor Frank Keating and United States Senator Don Nichols. Later, he spent a life-changing semester in Spain.

When Tyler was in his first year at Vanderbilt he called me one day and talked about how much family meant to him. He said I should not be surprised if he was married early in life. I teased him by suggesting that he might try dating first. He said he was just looking for a sweet girl.

Soon, he found the love of his life, a feisty, brilliant Italian girl from New Jersey, Elaine Marie Gulotta. It did not take them long to know they belonged together. I was thrilled with Elaine and her family, but not with the fact that I was losing Tyler to New Jersey. But what is a mother to do?

On May 29, 1999, Tyler married Elaine in Clinton, New Jersey, at a wedding that most girls dream of. While the wedding had Elaine's touch all over it, her parents had done much of the planning because Elaine was completing her degree at Vanderbilt where she graduated summa cum laude that spring. The wedding day and evening were among the most perfect days and nights of my life.

The actual wedding and reception were exceptionally beautiful. But the real success was based on the holiness of this union and the blessedness of the occasion. Love and laughter was poured out from every corner and created a river of joy that lifted us higher and higher.

One of my favorite scenes of the wedding was when I walked down the aisle as mother of the groom. I was escorted by my nephew, Jace. There were my dear friends and family who had been with me through thick and thin and had sacrificed their time and resources to come to New Jersey for this event. They knew what it meant to my heart to "give" Tyler up in marriage. I sat down in the pew and turned around and there were all my girlfriends with tears on their faces waving their hankies and Kleenexes at me in empathy. It was really dear and funny.

My friend, Connie McGoodwin, who has an only son who is younger, cried at every thing that happened. I told her she was my professional weeper and I would provide the same service for her when Colin, her son, was married.

Back at home, I believed Oklahomans should know how important the tourism industry was. I used a fable about a man looking for diamonds to convince citizens of the great worth of their local attractions. In the fable, a man leaves his home and travels all over the world looking for diamonds. When he finds none, he commits suicide. When his family assumed control of his farm, they found a huge diamond field in the back yard. There were diamonds there all the time. Oklahomans have diamonds in their back yards, as well—the parks, art museums, history, festivals and events, the water—we are a land rich with tourism treasures.

Governor Keating was very supportive of my leadership. I instituted his idea of a program called Oklahoma Overnight, in which we promoted visitors who were in the state for a particular conference or business trip to extend the trip one day, to take a road trip and see what we had to offer.

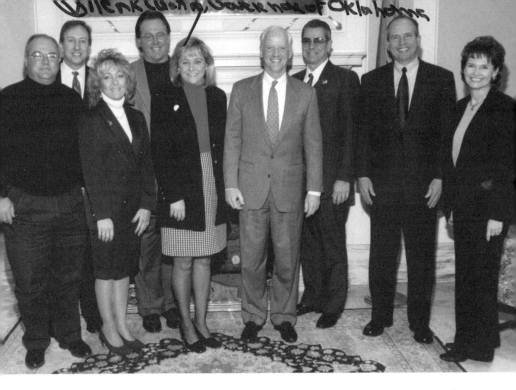

Above, the Oklahoma Tourism Commission oversees the operation of the agency. Left to right, front row, commissioner Boyd Lee, commissioner Janis Ricks, Lieutenant Governor Mary Fallin, Governor Frank Keating, commissioner Stan Clark, and me. Back row, assistant tourism director Doug Enevoldson, commissioner Hal Smith, and commissioner Joe Harwood. Commissioners not pictured were Robyn Batson and Joe Martin. Below, I joined Oklahoma First Lady Cathy Keating, left, and Arkansas First Lady Janet Huckabee, center, on a tour promoting tourism in western Arkansas and eastern Oklahoma.

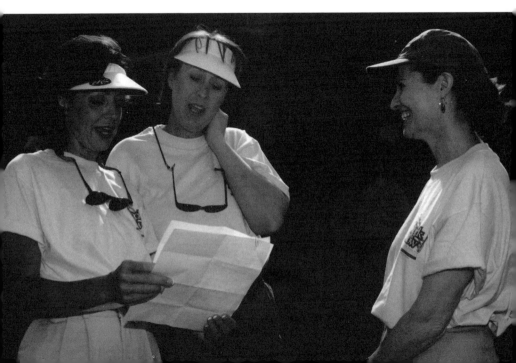

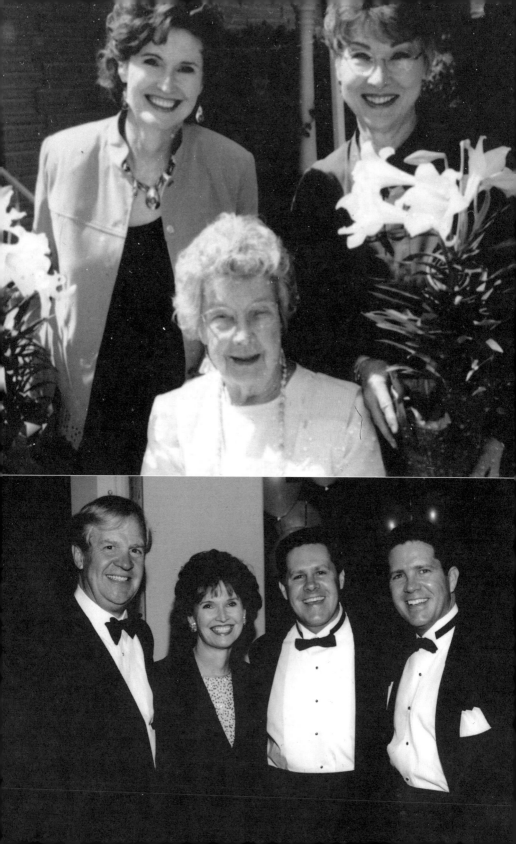

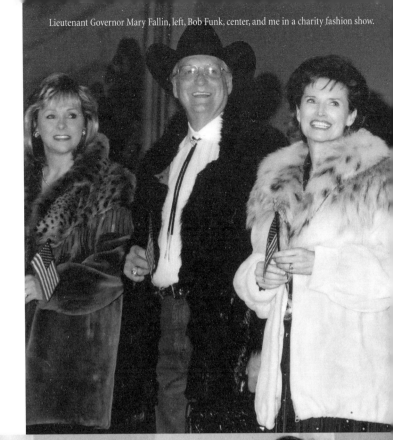

Lieutenant Governor Mary Fallin, left, Bob Funk, center, and me in a charity fashion show.

ft top, Mother, in front, and my
ster, Judy, right, have helped me
eather many storms in my life.
ft bottom, left to right, Jerry, me,
atch McCain, and Ben McCain,
others with whom I had worked
both Channel 4 and Channel 5.

elow, First Lady Cathy Keating,
ght, gave me great support as
ecretary of Tourism. She, and my
iend, Oklahoma Supreme Court
stice Yvonne Kauger, center, are
ole models for me.

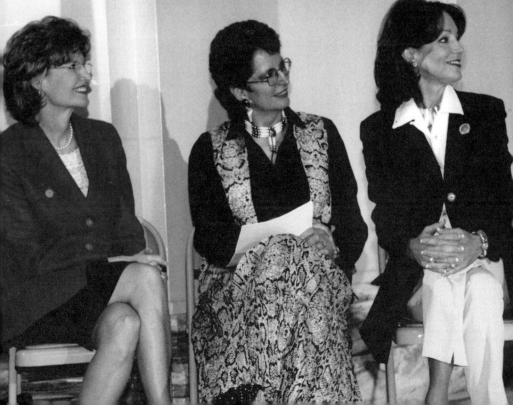

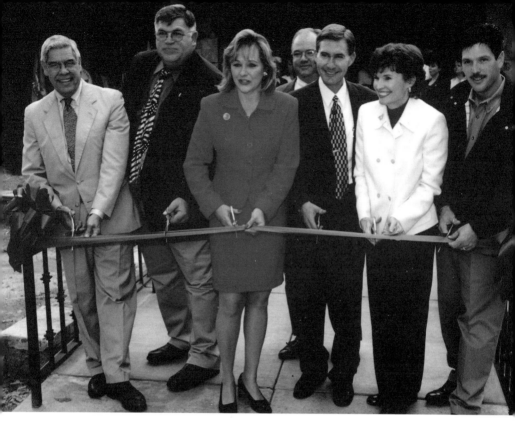

Left to right, Secretary of Transportation Neal McCaleb, State Senator Johnnie Crutchfield, Lieutenant Governor Mary Fallin, tourism commissioner Boyd Lee, State Representative Fred Stanley, me, and State Representative Greg Piatt. We were dedicating a new Oklahoma Welcome Center.

According to research, we were perceived as a poor, barren state, and I felt it was my job to make sure that every piece of promotional material told our real story as an exquisite place of beauty and recreational opportunity.

First Lady Cathy Keating was an amazing partner in promoting Oklahoma. She set up a tour of eastern Oklahoma and western Arkansas tourist spots with Arkansas First Lady Janet Huckabee. We canoed down the Illinois River together, rode horses, and visited several parks. The two first ladies promoted tourism at every stop—they had enormous energy and devotion to their roles, and they were kind to everyone and so much fun to be around. The promotion was such a success that we made plans for another trip the following fall.

The fall tour was to begin immediately after a highly promoted state tourism conference. However, during the conference, I received a call that my mother had suffered a severe stroke that had stilled the left side of her body.

I raced across the state to the hospital in Shattuck. Judy and I spent three days and nights with mother, taking our meals at the local Pizza Hut. I was so blessed to have an ever faithful sister like Judy. Daddy was at home—he was in very poor health. Mother had been full time caretaker for daddy for some time. He suffered one major health crisis after another. Mother and Judy were always there for him.

Mother was brought to Deaconess Hospital in Oklahoma City for five weeks of rehabilitation. My friend, Nancy Hall, PhD., was always on hand to help me make difficult medical decisions. I was so sad for my parents, growing old and facing tough times. Judy and I did our best to juggle our jobs and responsibilities to our parents. As usual, our extraordinary mother found humor in the hospital scene. When we would leave, we would say, "Okay, we'll be back." She would smile and respond, "Well, I'll be here!"

Even though Daddy was frail, Judy finally brought him to Deaconess Hospital to visit. There were tender times when we watched our parents, both in wheel chairs, show their love for each other that had nourished our lives. Mother was crying and Daddy was telling her how pretty she looked. When mother was sad about the terrible loss of ability she had suffered, I held her, paying her back for the thousands of times she had held me in her arms when I was hurt and afraid to go on with life.

I will never forget some of the moments in the hospital. There were times when mother was so sick and tired that her eyes would hardly focus. But, when I would get close and look at her, she would focus. When she saw me clearly, there would be so much love come into her eyes. She was an inspiration of courage to everyone, especially her therapists, and before long, she was bringing plum jelly from her Laverne kitchen to give away.

Judy and I got through the rehabilitation by assuring each other that the situation was not forever. Our theme was, "One day at a time." So many people were nice to us during the hospital stay. My parents had the most remarkable Laverne friends who helped. Bill Heaton and Walter Huffman checked on daddy at least once a day every day for many years. Clara Hartley has been our special angel and friend to mother as well as Dora Lujan. So many others showed the essence of Christian compassion.

I have learned a lot about being a friend from my parents whose lives were so wealthy in friends. People are always more important than politics. Friends laugh a lot, love each others' children, share pain, listen more than talk, and are always forgiving. My parents were selfless—and that goes a long way in cementing great relationships.

Judy has carried the bulk of the care for our parents, but we have shared many days and nights in hospital rooms during medical crises. One of the longest nights occurred in Shattuck. We know most of the nurses at that hospital because our parents had been admitted there so many times. We also knew and appreciated Dr. Flaherty, a remarkable doctor in a small, rural hospital. On a particular night, mother was having a bad time. Because of a bad reaction to medicine, she was extremely agitated and could not relax or be comforted. Judy and I took turns with her—then we tried singing to her. That seemed to help somewhat, so we sang about every song we knew. Toward morning, we just gave up and sat against the wall, numb to what was going on around us.

Then, we heard something. We opened our eyes and there were two nurses standing over mother's bed, singing to her. They were so precious. The next day, when mother improved, she thanked them and asked them to sing again. They laughed and said, "We'll never sing when you're in your right mind!"

I had great help promoting Oklahoma. The Ackerman McQueen advertising agency, and especially Peggy Howard, came up with innovative ways to display Oklahoma's assets. In partnership with the Oklahoma Travel Industry Association, the Oklahoma Hotel and Lodging Association, and the Oklahoma Restaurant Association, we launched an effort called Oklahoma's Newest Cash Crop, to show the importance of the tourism industry. Spending by tourists generated 67,000 jobs in Oklahoma and added nearly $4 billion dollars into the state's economy each year. My theme at speeches around the state was, "Tourism makes money for Oklahoma. Tourism generates jobs. Tourism is a sound investment. Investing more to sell our state develops our potential to clearly generate more profit."

Believe me, my job as tourism director was not all fun trips and speeches to grateful local citizens. It was difficult dealing with recalcitrant, politically motivated legislators. Chuck Ervin of the *Tulsa World* called my agency a "hotbed of patronage, politics, intramural blood letting, internal subterfuge, scheming, and backbiting."

In the agency, there were so many people who made my job a joy. My assistant, Leann Overstake, was heaven sent, as was deputy director, Doug Enevoldsen, who took on so much of the responsibility for legislative and financial issues that our complex agency faced daily. *Oklahoma Today* magazine had come a long way under the director of editor, Louisa McCune, from Enid. John Ressmeyer used his skills as a retired Marine colonel to professionalize our state park system. He was passionate about public land and an excellent administrator.

Because of John, we brought the National Association of State Park Directors annual conference to Oklahoma. Together with his deputy, Tom Creider, and my long time friend, Ron Stahl, the state park system greatly improved during those years. Jeff Erwin was a great hire from the private sector for our resorts division. Hardy Watkins was another fine addition to our marketing efforts in the travel and tourism division to work with Lori Nelson who had done an admirable job in reorganizing our publications and taking public relations efforts to a higher level. Amos Moses, Andrew Tevington, Betty Koehn, Gretchen Harris, Kris Marek, Joan Henderson, Craig Sanger, Larry Habegger, Dino Lalli, Kathlean Marks, Sandy Pantlik, and so many others formed an outstanding team. And, as a member of the governor's cabinet, I interacted with brilliant state leaders and worked closely with several of them such as Russell Perry, Neal McCaleb, Howard Barnett, Tom Daxon, Oscar Jackson, and Bob Ricks.

The role of the Tourism Commission, chaired by the lieutenant governor, is extremely important. Thanks to Governor Keating and Kay Dudley, we had an incredibly fine commission. There were experts from the tourism industry, successful men and women of integrity who were willing to be bold and brave when it came to making tough decisions for the departments within the agency.

Not only was our group of commissioners well respected in the industry, and among the leading professionals in the state, they were fun and caring human beings who left the agency in better shape than they found it.

As much as I enjoyed the people with whom I worked daily in the Colcord Building in Oklahoma City, I have to say that one of my greatest rewards was to meet the men and women who worked in the field. The people who were stationed at state parks were totally dedicated to the importance of public land for all people—for all time. Our regional managers were well educated, dedicated family men who usually lived on the property and really took care of everything.

An example of the dedication of our employees was made evident when my husband and I stopped at a remote state park in the Oklahoma Panhandle on our way to Colorado. It was a Sunday morning but the park director and his wife were out working. No other employees were available on Sunday because of the agency's reduced budget, so the director and his non-state-employee wife were filling in. I cannot say enough good things about these employees.

FRANK KEATING

~ ~ ~ *"One of my most brilliant moves as governor of Oklahoma was to appoint Jane Secretary of Tourism. Her love for Oklahoma and great ability to promote our many recreation opportunities made her a valued member of my cabinet."*

CATHY KEATING

~ ~ ~ *"Never in my wildest dreams did I think I would ever meet Jane, much less come to know her as a dear friend. I was one of the millions of teenaged girls watching as she was crowned Miss America. It was not until Frank became governor that I learned that my teenage idol's beauty and poise ran deeper than her skin.*

As I suspected, there was much more strength of character, determination, and perseverance, a mirror of "pioneer woman." She is a smart and respected leader, but the Jane I admire and love is loyal, caring, and loving. In my book, 40 years later, she still wears a crown."

KIRK HUMPHREYS

~ ~ ~ *"Jane is a beauty—no secret there! As I got to know her, I discovered that her inner person is where the true beauty lies. Jane cares about people—those who are important in the world's eyes, and those who are not—those who are physically attractive, and those who are not—those who are wealthy and famous, and those who are poor and invisible. When Jane looks upon a person with her beautiful blue eyes, every person—big or small—feels important. Jane sees people as God sees them—with love, grace, forgiveness, and hope."*

KAY DUDLEY

~ ~ ~ *"Jane is a sensitive, caring, and deeply spiritual lady. To say that she is talented, modest, gentle, and unassuming seems overly complimentary but it is too true not to mention. If I am ever stranded on a desert island it would be great to have Jane there with me. "*

BOB RICKS

~ ~ ~ *"I had the pleasure of getting to know Jane when we were both members of Governor Frank Keating's cabinet. I cannot think of a single meeting where by her mere presence she did not lift the spirits of everyone and always projected a humble caring spirit. Whenever we traveled throughout the state, everyone knew Jane and pressed to shake her hand and get a moment of her time. She handled every encounter with class and grace— everyone was treated with kindness and gentleness, and everyone with whom she visited was made to feel special."*

STEVEN E. MOORE

~ ~ ~ *"Her awards and talents have enabled Jane to do a magnificent job of representing our state and presenting it in the best possible way. I recall an Oklahoma City Chamber of Commerce reception in Jane and Jerry's home. The high point of the evening was when Jane stepped to their grand piano in their living room and performed several songs. Our gathering was transformed into a special and very personal, world-class musical performance by a former Miss America, rivaling entertainment in any venue, anywhere. Jane absolutely held everyone's full attention and affection. I remember thinking, "Jane is truly a treasure of this state!"*

RUSSELL PERRY

~ ~ ~ *"It was a joy to serve on Governor Keating's cabinet with Jane. She brought her love for Oklahoma to the table, and we were all better for it."*

DOUG ENEVOLDSEN

~ ~ ~ *"She is a living example of the noble characteristic of grace. As Director of Tourism, she faced many challenges of dealing with the realities of politics. During a scathing attack from an unhappy legislator, she was wonderful, showing courage, class, and grace under fire. She stood her ground and made a principled, courageous decision. She led an effort to establish priorities within the state parks system and raised awareness of the decaying condition of state facilities. She was proud to promote the state which she so dearly loves."*

LEANN OVERSTAKE

~ ~ ~ *"As her executive assistant at the Department of Tourism, I witnessed first hand Jane's true leader qualities and her quest for excellence. God gave her exquisite beauty and filled her with grace. Her parents instilled in her qualities of integrity, determination, and kindness."*

JOHN RESSMEYER

~ ~ ~ *"As Secretary of Tourism Jane's unique personality allowed her to bridge the perceived gap between staff/employees in the field and headquarters staff in Oklahoma City. She was always available to meet with park employees and displayed a genuine interest in each state park. There was no doubt she was intelligent, insightful, and knowledgeable about the agency's priorities and goals."*

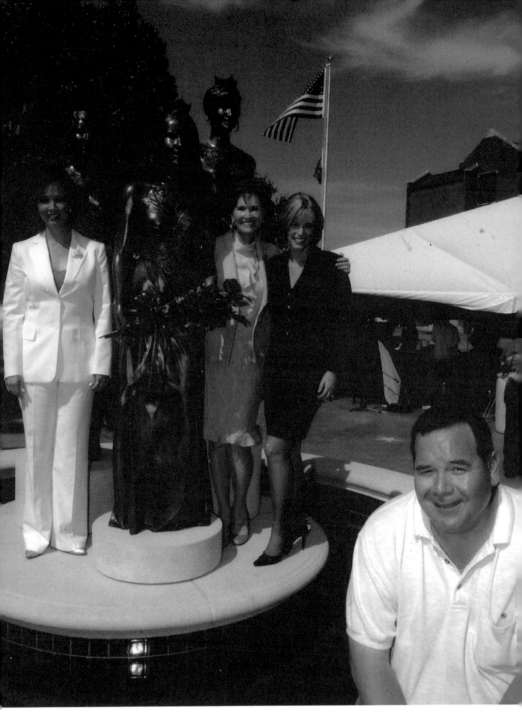

In the spring of 2005, Oklahoma City University dedicated the sculpture honoring OCU's three Miss Americas. Edward L. Gaylord provided funding for the larger-than-life bronze. My heart was overflowing as I stood with Susan Powell, left, and Shawntel Smith Wuerch, right, at the dedication of the sculpture. In the forefront is sculptor, Shan Gray, of Edmond, Oklahoma.

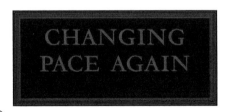

20

CHANGING
PACE AGAIN

*O*ne of the challenges in running the state's tourism program was using money wisely. Our state parks system had been under funded for many years. When disasters such as the fire that destroyed Quartz Mountain State Lodge near Altus occurred, more budget problems followed. In 2000, a Christmas ice storm left more than $2 million damage and cleanup costs in state parks. Many areas of Beavers Bend State Park were decimated by the weight of ice on trees, some of which were 50 years old. I was so proud of parks department personnel who worked night and day for weeks to reopen Beavers Bend to the public. Robbers Cave State Park and even some of the western state parks were also hard hit by the ice.

Governor Keating was aware of our plight and supported increased budgets during my tenure as tourism director. He always made time for cabinet members to keep him abreast of what was happening on their watch. Some of my favorite times in government were quick lunches when the governor was inspirational, urging cabinet members to hurry, because the time of his administration was ticking away.

While I was traveling around the state and keeping up with a busy schedule, my sister, Judy, was spending more time than ever taking care of our parents. On an icy night in late 2000, she had to rush mother to the hospital. The roads were so bad, I could not drive to western Oklahoma.

I sat and thought how I had really failed these women, the two best human beings in the world. That night, I dreamed mother had died. The dream was so real, that when I called the hospital the next morning, I expected them to tell me that she was no longer alive. Fortunately, I was wrong. When I talked to mother, she related a dream she had. She was on

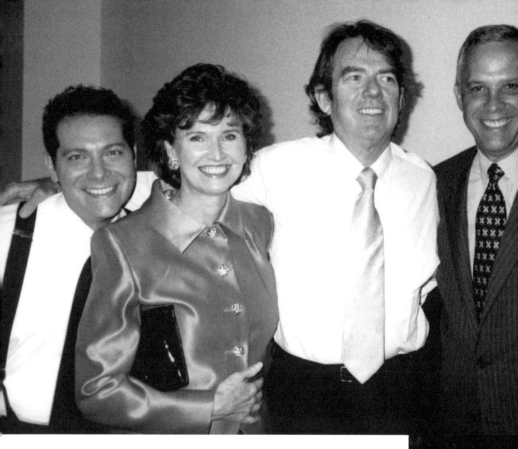

At the opening of the renovated Civic Center Music Hall in Oklahoma City are, left to right, Michael Feinstein, me, Jimmy Webb, and Oklahoma City Mayor Kirk Humphreys. Right, Oklahomans streamed onto Broadway to walk to the theater for the opening of "Oklahoma!" Left to right, Oklahoma City Mayor Kirk Humphreys, former Governor George Nigh, former First Lady Donna Nigh, First Lady Cathy Keating, Governor Frank Keating. Jerry and I are behind the Keatings.

It was a gala occasion at the dedication of the State Capitol dome in November, 2002. Left to right, Susan Powell, Shawntel Smith Wuerch, me, and singer Vince Gill.

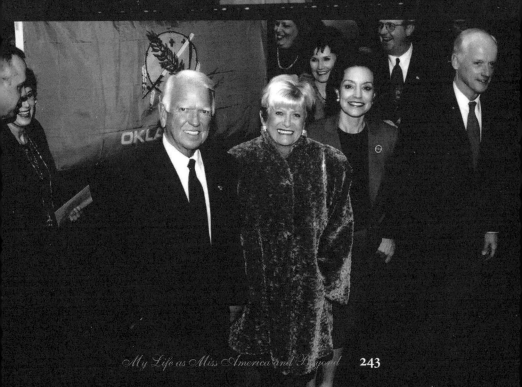

stage at a pageant in Laverne when her deceased sister, in a beautiful, flowing white gown, walked to the front of the auditorium and touched mother. Then she went to the back to wait.

I believe mother almost died that night, but God gave her back her life so she could stay with daddy until his death just a month later. He would have been so miserable without her. Daddy died peacefully on January 21, 2001—he just did not wake up one morning. It was a perfect answer to our prayers after all he had been through. In one of God's many graces, we were all together at home the night daddy died. Mother has done exceedingly well since daddy's death. She determined in her heart that even though she was in a wheel chair, she would be independent, would adjust to life, and make the most of what she has been given.

After we said goodbye to daddy, it was back to work for me. If politicians were not taking pot shots at me, the agency had some financial crisis. Daddy's death had left me in a delicate condition, so I took more time to make decisions. Often when a huge decision needed to be made, I took an extra breath and moved on. I believed I created a positive atmosphere for the tourism industry in Oklahoma.

In March, 2002, I led a delegation of Oklahoma leaders to New York City for opening night of the revival of *Oklahoma!* on Broadway. Lee Allan Smith helped me raise funds from private sources so the state could participate in this historic occasion. Governor Keating and First Lady Cathy Keating led the delegation along with former Governor George Nigh and former First Lady Donna Nigh.

We generated an enormous amount of publicity for opening night. We had an Oklahoma trick roper and Guthrie's Byron Berline, an incredible musician. CNN Headline News showed all day the delegation walking down Broadway to the theater. It was such an uplifting and positive news story after all Oklahoma and New York City had been through in the post 9-11 days. Governor Keating was a popular political figure in New York City and there was genuine excitement in the air about the musical.

In addition to the many Oklahomans who flew in for the event, we invited some friends in New York City from Oklahoma to join us. Jimmy Webb, Bill and Barbara Geddie, former Miss America Susan Powell, and OCU graduate and Broadway star Kristen Chenoweth were there. I worked with

Bill and Barbara at Channel 5 in 1978. Bill now produces television shows such as "The View" and Barbara Walters' specials. A lot of other famous people attended the opening night festivities, including Barbara Walters, Donald Trump, Shirley Jones, and Oklahoma film stars Rue McClanahan and Tony Randall.

There was a lot of excitement during my four years at tourism. In spite of enormous problems, we managed to get Quartz Mountain Arts and Conference Center opened after many delays. Also, the beautiful 18-hole golf course at Lake Texoma, Chickasaw Pointe, opened. Nine holes were added to the Roman Nose State Park golf course. A beautiful Welcome Center was built and opened near the Texas border at Thackerville. We decorated it with the help of many Oklahoma City and Norman area museums that provided art work to encourage visitors to see their museums.

Welcome Centers were also opened outside Tulsa to cover Claremore and other northeastern cities, and at Colbert and Sallisaw. According to a poll, the image of tourism in Oklahoma had a huge positive increase around this time and I know we made a difference.

On May 25, 2002, I became a grandmother. Elaine gave birth to Luke Michael Jayroe. He was the most beautiful baby in the world with lots of black hair. All I could think about was Tyler being a baby, and how God had seen us through the bad times to bring us to this cherished hour. I kept wondering, "How can I sing loud enough to express to God my gratitude for Luke?"

When Brad Henry was elected governor in November, 2002, I suspected my days as tourism director might be numbered. After all, I had been appointed by a Republican governor and Governor Henry was a Democrat. I respected a new governor's right to have his own people in key state agency positions, although I would have loved to continue to lead Oklahoma's efforts to tell the whole world what a wonderful place the Sooner State is.

The week after the election, I appeared with OCU's two other Miss Americas, Susan Powell and Shawntell Smith Wuerch, Vince Gill, Amy Grant, Leona Mitchell, Jimmy Webb, and other celebrities at the dedication of the new dome atop the State Capitol in Oklahoma City. Lee Allan Smith orchestrated what has to be one of the grandest celebrations Oklahoma has ever seen. I was so proud of Oklahoma that night!

Shortly after the Henry administration took over in January, 2003, it was obvious that I would be replaced. I accepted that fact as a political reality and moved on. However, it was heartbreaking for me to see so many other tourism people lose their jobs in the transition.

In 2004, I became the national spokesperson for Oklahoma City University's centennial celebration. It gave me an opportunity to give back to the university and work with OCU President Tom and Brenda McDaniel, longtime friends from Laverne and Alva.

One of the projects of which I had dreamed was in the distance on my radar screen. During my friendship with Kay Dudley, who was a Christian mentor to me, she often quoted from the book of Esther in the Bible during times I was discouraged or feeling inept. Kay told me I was created, just like Esther, "for a time like this."

If those words were such a great encouragement to me, I thought, surely other women needed the teaching. Maybe God was calling me to take the

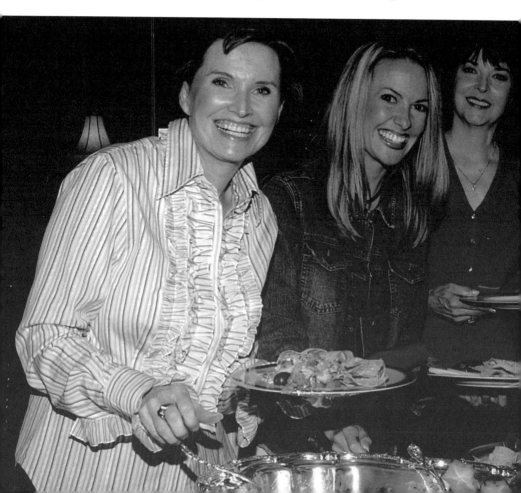

elow left, former Miss Oklahomas joined me
r dinner at an Oklahoma City University
ntennial celebration. Left to right, Kelli
asters, Beverly Hoster, and Jill Patton. Right,
e best part of being honored by OCU
ocieties was sharing the event with inspiring
llow honorees and friends. Left to right,
anda Bass, me, and Sue Hale, and Beth
olbert.

am privileged to be one of the three Miss
mericas who attended Oklahoma City
niversity—surely a record in the Miss
merica Pageant. Left to right, Susan Powell,
iss America 1981, Shawntel Smith Wuerch,
iss America 1996, and me.

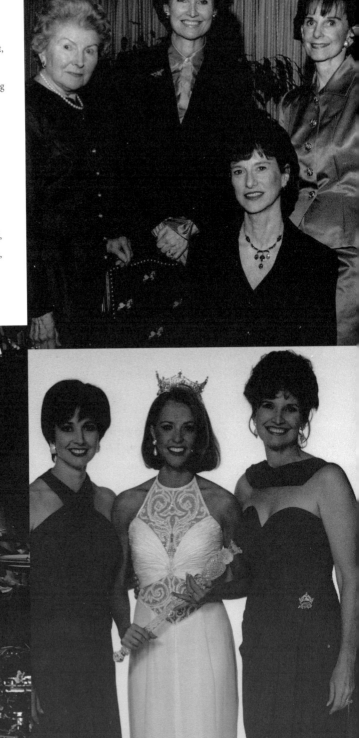

message to other busy women. I created a six-week class for women titled, "Esther Women: created for such a time as this." I offered the class at Oklahoma City University and invited some of my favorite women to attend and to help me teach the class. Teachers and table hosts who participated in that first effort were Reverend Linda Brinkworth, Bobbie Roe, LaDonna Meinders, Cathy Leichter, Kay Dudley, Connie McGoodwin, Dr. Lori Hansen, Barbara Green, and Brenda McDaniel.

Esther Women is now an ongoing faith development-friendship building experience that is monthly in nature and blessed by many special and beautiful women. It has been a labor of love!

Two of the big events I was able to work on for OCU brought great personal rewards. For the Celebration of the Century, I worked with Lee Allan Smith, Bill Thrash, and Silvertree Productions. OCU invited all former students who had held the Miss Oklahoma title or other state title to appear in a style show sponsored by the OCU Societies and Balliets. President Tom McDaniel and his wife, Brenda, hosted a lovely dinner for the girls.

The following morning was the official dedication of the Miss America statues, a perfect fall day to honor the three OCU students, Susan Powell, Shawntel Smith Wuerch, and me, who have won the Miss America crown. OCU alumnus Chris Harrison, host of "The Bachelor" and the Miss America Pageant, was our master of ceremonies. Kerr McGee Corporation president Luke Corbett led the dedication of the Kerr McGee Park on the campus. The entire student body of the music school performed an original piece of music, "Cradle of Dreams" by Edward Knight, text by M.J. Alexander. It was a holy moment!

Lee Allan had produced a huge crown covering the statue of the three Miss Americas. With a drum roll and countdown from the audience, the crown was pulled apart and balloons escaped into the air. It was a lovely moment for Susan, Shawntel, and me, and the 15 other Miss Oklahoma's who walked over to join in the celebration. What a tradition LaDonna Meinders began for OCU when she was named Miss Oklahoma in 1956. She was the first of 33 state title holders and three Miss Americas from OCU.

Another rewarding event for me at OCU was a communications conference we produced for the spring of 2005. I had dreamed of staging something at OCU to draw students interested in journalism and have them hear

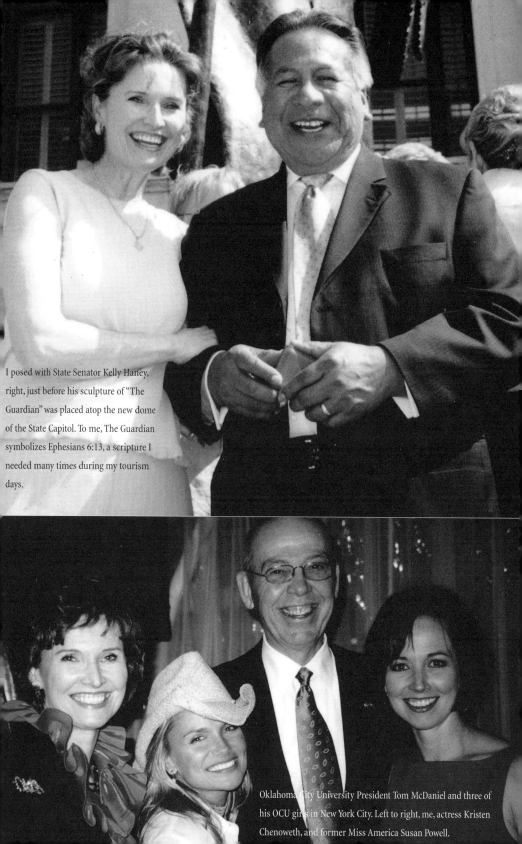

I posed with State Senator Kelly Haney, right, just before his sculpture of "The Guardian" was placed atop the new dome of the State Capitol. To me, The Guardian symbolizes Ephesians 6:13, a scripture I needed many times during my tourism days.

Oklahoma City University President Tom McDaniel and three of his OCU girls in New York City. Left to right, me, actress Kristen Chenoweth, and former Miss America Susan Powell.

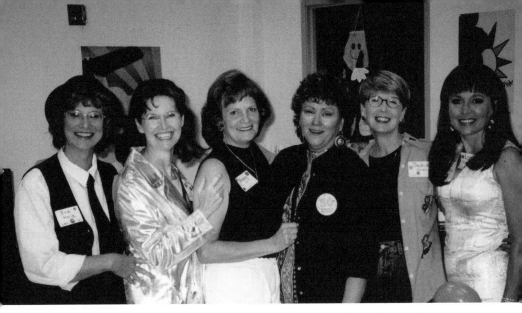

Members of my Facets group at a costume party. Left to right, Sue Hale, me, Nancy Hall, Connie McGoodwin, Jackie Jones, and Dr. Lori Hansen. All of us love to laugh!

Karen Hughes, who had become a familiar face on American television. Karen is considered to be President Bush's closest advisor on all communications issues and had just been appointed Under Secretary of State. Karen and I had worked together at KXAS in Dallas.

Thanks to the Ethics and Excellence in Journalism Foundation, we were able to bring Karen to the campus. The Oklahoma City Community Foundation provided funds to buy lunch for nearly 800 journalism students from across Oklahoma who participated in the great day of discussion about ethics in political journalism.

We had an impressive panel, including two of my best friends, Sue Hale and Linda Cavanaugh. We also brought in Ken Bode, the former PBS moderator of "Week in Review" and former dean of the journalism school at Northwestern University.

Karen helped make the day a huge success. She was tireless. She met with OCU communications students after the conference at the president's home. Then she spoke at a fund raising dinner that evening. We were able to raise $100,000 for the first ever scholarship for mass communications at OCU. We named it in honor of a beautiful young woman, Brooke Haley, who had recently died from cancer. Brooke was a former Miss OCU and an

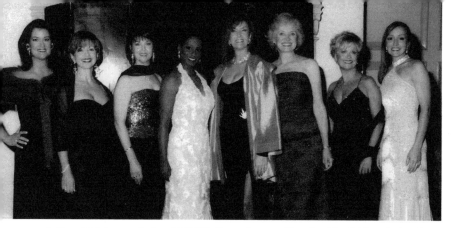

LaDonna Meinders was the first of 33 OCU ladies to win a state title such as Miss Oklahoma in the Miss America system. These eight former Miss Oklahomas helped celebrate the OCU Centennial. Left to right, Mignon Merchant Ball, Jill Elmore Patton, Beverly Drew Hoster, DuSharme Llanusa Carter, Debbi Giannopoulus Mustafoglu, LaDonna Kramer Meinders, Debbie Knight, and Kristen Steveson Schriks.

outstanding communications student. Her death was such a tragedy, but this honor was something everyone felt she would have loved.

Life is amazingly full and enjoyable for me. I have the opportunity to serve my community in a variety of volunteer efforts including the board of trustees of the Oklahoma City Community Foundation, Church of the Servant, and Oklahoma City University. Thanks to Speaker of the House Todd Hiett, I can continue to serve Oklahoma by participating on the Oklahoma Centennial Commission.

I have wonderful friends—some lifelong, some new friends. I always have room for a new girlfriend. As I age, my women friends are even more important. They bring a sense of laughter to life that is so important and we kind of "mother" each other as our own parents have moved into a different role. Besides, I need them to remember things.

One of my gifts has been to be able to successfully bring women together. After that, they form bonds, and when God is part of the process, there is something far deeper that occurs. In addition to my lifelong friends, church friends, work friends, and family, I put together a group of women known as "Facets" about 1990. We have become sisters in a deep and caring way. Through joint travel, birthday celebrations, the sharing of our awards and joys, as well as our deepest griefs, we have forged a profound bond. The group is amazingly competent without being competitive. We serve as a professional resource for each other, an ever present help in times of trouble, and the encouraging voice that is needed even among the most accomplished of our group. The group consists of Sue Hale, executive editor of *The Daily Oklahoman,* Connie Thrash McGoodwin, director of the Dale Rogers Training Center, Nancy Hall, PhD., associate dean of the OU College of Medicine, Dr. Lori Hansen Lane, facial plastic surgeon, and Jackie Jones, former Oklahoma City Arts Council director and currently director of Turning Point. We have all blazed trails in our own ways, and yet in the midst of being so responsible, manage to be really goofy when we are together. What a huge blessing it is to have a group of people in which there exists total trust, a penchant to silliness, and an absolute knowledge that whatever comes our way, we will be there for each other in very practical and personal ways.

Good friends and a solid family help give life a proper perspective. When my nephew, Dal, was a senior at Laverne High School, he teased me about Main Street being named Jane Jayroe Boulevard. He said it was really neat—instead of dragging Main, he and his friends dragged Jane! Kids are humbling! If I were to give advice to another young person who was suddenly thrust into the opportunity of a lifetime, at the top of my list would be to surround yourself with trusted friends and family who tell you the truth, love you—but do not adore you—and people who help you laugh even at yourself. My greatest blessings are in friends and family.

I try to practice what I preach—choose an attitude of grace about life. The apostle Paul writes a lot about the importance of "joy" and how we find it even in the dark times of life. In fact, he says to count it all joy—I'm beginning to understand what he means. God can bring something good out of every situation. My mother models that every day of her life.

If I had never been divorced, I would not be married to Jerry Gamble today. If I had not been desperate for money as a single mother, I would never have found a career that was incredibly satisfying. If I had not faced a demotion in television because of my return to Oklahoma, I would never have worked with the Presbyterian Health Foundation and Oklahoma Health Center. All of these "failures" led to wonderful opportunities, including serving on Governor Keating's cabinet.

Living an unexpected life by accepting grace, living with grit, and loving with a grateful heart is a blessing beyond description.

REVEREND LINDA BRINKWORTH

~ ~ ~ *"Jane has a countenance of calm while still firmly grounded in reality. More importantly, Jane is a person of impeccable integrity, humor, honesty, and humility. She is consistent, whether in the public eye or in private friendships."*

BARBARA GREEN

~ ~ ~ *"Jane is a glamorous woman, but much more than that. She is full of grace, a gentle person who, in spite of her notoriety, is approachable and attentive to others. She is a mover and a shaker, even in her gentleness. She is a deeply spiritual and compassionate leader for our state and nation."*

SUE HALE

~ ~ ~ *"I admire Jane's sense of humor and her willingness to listen and share her own thoughts on any topic. True friends give you unconditional love and support and Jane is a true friend. I am proud of her passion for Oklahoma. When she was tourism director, she insisted we take a field trip to Quartz Mountain. On a hike, we were sweating and swatting bugs, but Jane was forging ahead with enthusiasm. And when we stopped to rest and look around us, she was right—Oklahoma is beautiful.*

The most important lesson I have learned from Jane is that beauty on the inside is more important than a pretty face. That might sound strange since she is a former Miss America. But she knows that what is in your heart determines who you really are and how you live your life is how you will be remembered."

~ ~ ~ *"Jane's relationship with Christ provides a foundation for most of the close friendships six women share in a group called "Facets" that Jane created in 1990 as a support group for professional women. Jackie Jones, Connie Thrash McGoodwin, Lori Hansen Lane, Sue Hale, and I represent all facets of life and life's challenges. Our group of women is prayerful, supportive, and shares all the sorrows and challenges of growing older definitely with more grace than glamour.*

We began as individuals in a morning prayer group focused on making it through each day with some balance and grace. We celebrated birthdays, even the big ones ending in zeroes at exotic places like Branson, Missouri, rejoiced in community awards and honors for each other, and shared sorrows and disappointments of every day occurrences in our lives and those of our children and families."

MICK CORNETT

~ ~ ~ *"Meeting Jane many years ago in our early television days was like walking into a fairy tale and running into the princess. She was polite, courteous, on-time, and very curious. Even though she had a lot to learn, she was willing to work hard to shorten the learning curve."*

PHYLLIS GEORGE

~ ~ ~ *"I met Jane when I was competing for the Miss Texas title. Jane was the emcee. Somehow we connected and I felt as though she was secretly rooting for me the night I won.*

Jane has always been one of my favorite Miss Americas because of her intelligence, beauty, and elegance. She has been a role model for many young women. Her generosity of spirit and gracious ways continue to inspire me."

254

~ ~ ~ *"In 2003, Jane organized a Bible study to meet at
Oklahoma City University, calling on her many friends, from
housewives to judges, educators, and various other fields. The
group, which first studied the book of Esther, became fondly
known as "Esther women," even to the point of our seeing a
fellow member at any event and embracing one another as
"Esther sisters." Jane is a unique person to be able to draw a
diverse group of women into this kind of closeness, and now we
don't want the study to ever end. Through all Jane's important
awards and honors, she has a heart for Oklahoma, a true
Christian spirit, appreciation of her friends and colleagues, and a
remarkable humility to go along with her confident leadership. I
am honored to call her my friend."*

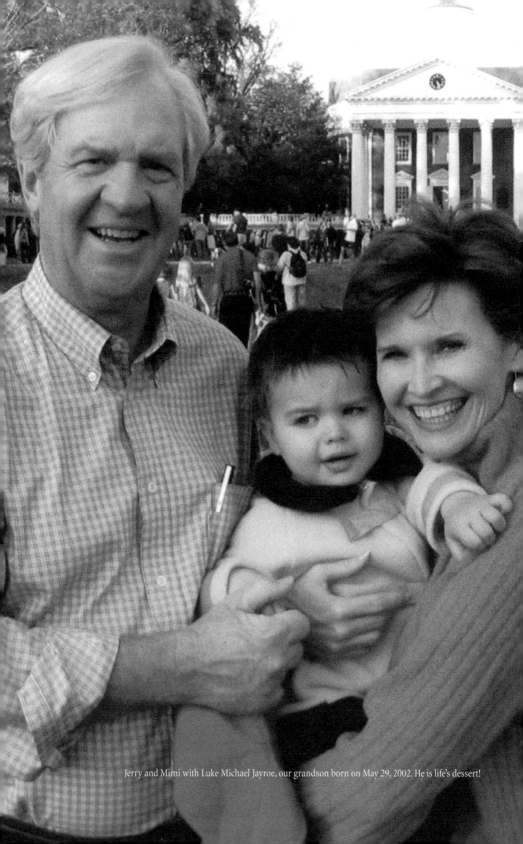
Jerry and Mimi with Luke Michael Jayroe, our grandson born on May 29, 2002. He is life's dessert!

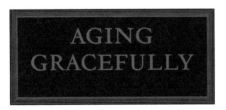

21

AGING
GRACEFULLY

*I*t has been four decades since I walked the runway as Miss America and over ten years since my final broadcast as a television news anchor. Several years ago, on a trip to Salt Lake City, I noticed that people do not look at me anymore. It had been happening gradually, but I had not noticed it until that moment—in airports, restaurants, at the mall—no one looks at me anymore. While that seems unimportant in the overall scheme of life, it was a different experience for me because my career had always been linked to personal appearance. Oh sure, I could still turn a head if I was dressed up for a special occasion and went to a lot of work. But in regular circumstances, I was one of the crowd—a bit different for me.

My history is framed with attention. I began entering beauty pageants when I was a senior in high school. While winning titles as Miss Oklahoma City, Miss Oklahoma, and Miss America, I could not avoid being looked at. It was as if a neon sign was hanging over my head, demanding attention. The crown, the banners, the fanfare, the sign on the side of the car all announced me. The attention was so great at times that I needed body-guards. Even when I traveled anonymously, bystanders often stared.

After the pageant years, when my career turned to broadcast journalism, the public's recognition of me skyrocketed. For 17 years I was nightly in the homes of millions of people. At that time, I could hardly walk across the street without someone asking, "Aren't you Jane Jayroe?" or "Did anyone ever tell you that you look a lot like Jane Jayroe?" Almost everywhere I went,

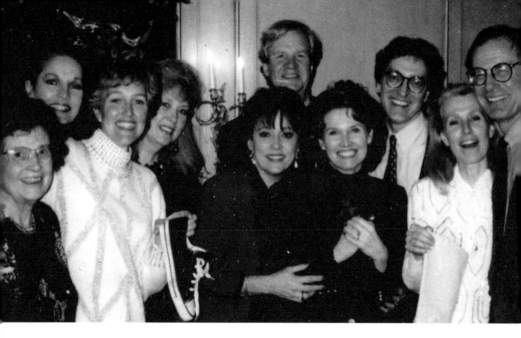

I could feel the looks directed my way. Usually they were just curious stares—not intrusive or rude, but nonetheless direct.

After my retirement from television, the recognition gradually faded. I began asking questions of myself, "Who will I be if I am no longer one of the pretty ones or that lady on the news?"

In some ways this is a time of life I had grown to fear. Remember the sad image of a fading rose, a pitiful metaphor for a "has-been?" I once wept in a London theater when I saw the musical *Sunset Boulevard*. In a powerful scene, the aging actress comes back to the movie studio because she believes she can recapture her former grandeur and success. But in the glare of reality, she appears foolish and out of touch. She sits totally wilted on a stool in the center of the stage. Then, something magical happens?

The huge lights turn on—spotlights from all directions illuminate her like a life source from heaven. People look at her, applauding, and the music swells. The former leading lady blooms like a flower, right in front of the eyes of the people in the audience. At long last the eccentric actress, like a wilted and dying plant, is given light and water from above. She grows and regains life and sings from the depths of her being.

What a theatrical moment! But after the moment, after the applause, the light on the stage fades. It was artificial. The life-giving energy dissipates, as

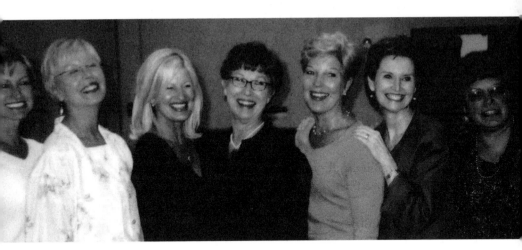

glamour often does, and the final result is devastating for the actress. I wept with the power of the moment and empathy for the character. I knew about that spotlight from a different position. I understood that attention can be addictive and false images can become so powerful that they become who you are, and not simply a role you play. You can end a successful career as a lonely, sad person, whose only claim in life is a "former" something.

When the moment in Salt Lake City hit me, I felt relief. It was okay not to be noticed. It was convenient to fit into a crowd. I had no intention of being powerless or invisible, but I knew that I mattered not because of the attention I received, but because of the people I loved and by the God I served. After an entire lifetime seeking fame and success, I was comfortable being out of the spotlight. I was not Miss America or "that lady on the news," but I was Janie Jayroe from the plains of Oklahoma—the person God created from the inside out. I knew that by the grace of God, my future was just as great a gift as my past—just different. "Being confident of this, that He who began a good work in you (and me) will go on to perfect it until the day of Christ Jesus." Philippians 1:6. God clearly has much work to do on me.

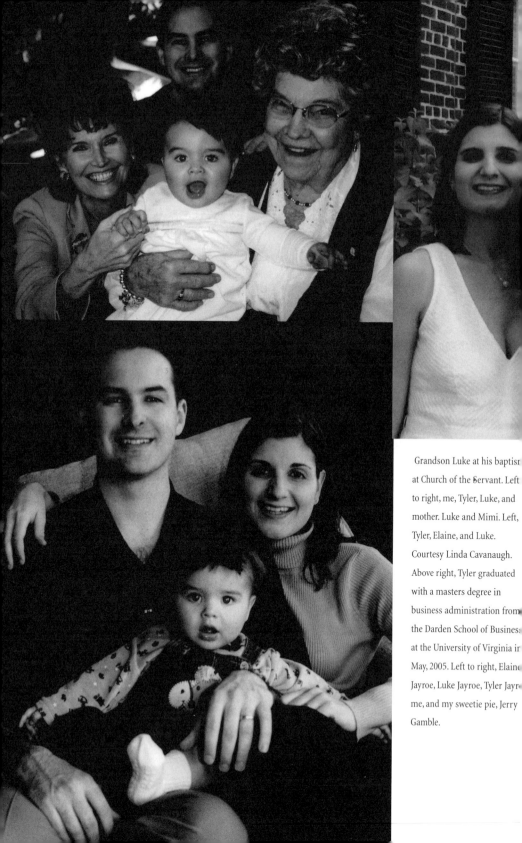

Grandson Luke at his baptism at Church of the Servant. Left to right, me, Tyler, Luke, and mother. Luke and Mimi. Left, Tyler, Elaine, and Luke. Courtesy Linda Cavanaugh. Above right, Tyler graduated with a masters degree in business administration from the Darden School of Business at the University of Virginia in May, 2005. Left to right, Elaine Jayroe, Luke Jayroe, Tyler Jayroe, me, and my sweetie pie, Jerry Gamble.

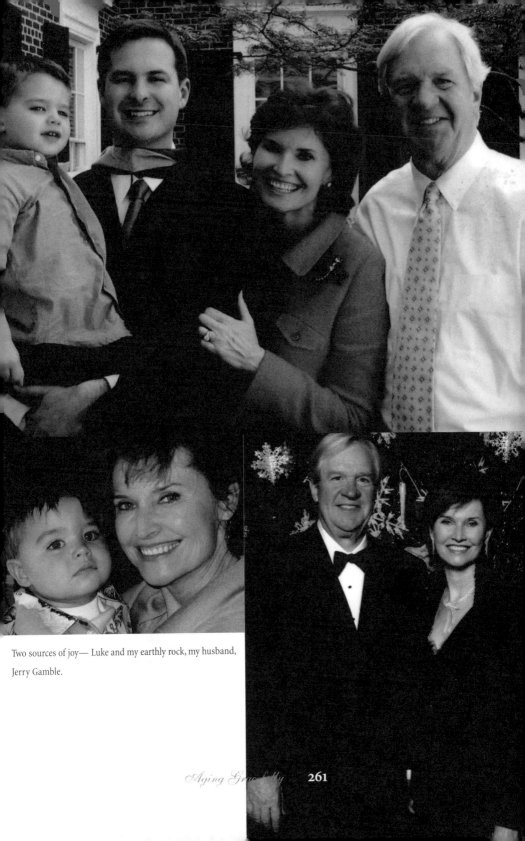

Two sources of joy— Luke and my earthly rock, my husband, Jerry Gamble.

As I try to age gracefully—in God's grace—my perspective is no longer from the starring role. I now take comfort in the journey thus far and give thanks for all of it. There will be new challenges and different chapters ahead and I pray that I will give out in service rather than sit out in retirement.

I have lived through valleys and heartaches, but also have been blessed with some peak moments few people will ever know—walking the runway the length of a football field with spotlights aglow and standing crowds applauding, performing for thousands of servicemen in Vietnam, and meeting some of the most important people on earth.

Most importantly, I still have me after all the applause has hushed and lights dimmed. Because I have tried to live my life as a child of god, those things that really matter—loving the Lord and learning to walk with him—have grown stronger with time. His presence inside of me keeps me grounded. I can enjoy the sparkles of life without becoming seduced by them. I find a tomorrow when the light of today fades. Realizing that God makes us from the inside out seems to me to be crucial in managing the turns of life's journey. I believe that God blesses our struggles in the process.

So as I turn this curve in my life, I think of others who have had their day in the sun—athletes, politicians, rock stars, coaches, movie stars, business leaders, and pretty young people. We have been blessed that our journey has had highs. If we are centered in our faith, the journey does not end when the highs fade away. We simply move from one phase of life to another. But if we do not make the transition, if we have become addicted to the attention of yesterday, we become an object of pity. We become the person who wilts in the light of day and can shine only once in a while with an artificial source. God designed us for the true light and prepares us for the road ahead if we will let Him.

Writing this book with Bob Burke has been an amazing experience. Retracing my life has caused me to wince with shame at my mistakes and feel my heart squeeze in pain at the loss of loved ones. But primarily I have been overwhelmed by how blessed my life has been. During the work on the book, two incidents occurred that touched me deeply about my journey.

It was a hot summer day when I visited a man who fits me for orthotics—those pageant shoes are destructive. We were talking about everything when he asked, "Are you still head of tourism?" I told him, "No," that the governor had wanted a different person in the job, and that was fine with me. I loved tourism, but it was also fine to move on to the next chapter of my life. He lowered his head and said that some time back he and his wife had lost their son. When life overwhelmed them, they visited our state parks. He said that anytime they were at a park, they thought of me. He said, "If you ever get a chance, please tell those folks who work in the parks how much they mean to people like us."

By the time he ended his story, I had big tears in my eyes and a lump in my throat.

A few weeks earlier, I was having lunch with my friend, Cathy Leichter. Her brother, who was serving in Vietnam when I was there as Miss America, had found a 1967 *Oklahoma Today* magazine that had my photograph on the cover. Even though he hardly ever asked Cathy for anything, he did request that she get the magazine signed by me. I was humbled because it meant so much to him that I had gone to Vietnam.

I do not know why I have been given such an incredible gift of being able to matter to people. What a privilege! It is not deserved nor earned. I have been given so much and forgiven so much, for my life's journey is littered with poor judgment, harsh words, unnecessary criticism, and mistakes. I have never desired to be on a pedestal—it distances you from people, and it is too easy to fall off. It is enough to try to live a good life day by day—some times are better than others. This I do know, and would stake my life on—God is good. Blessings abound! Oklahoma is as much a part of me as my own skin.

God has granted me grace through Jesus Christ. It is not because of something I did, but because of who He is. It has been fun to have some glamorous years, but real joy has come from an abundant and amazing grace. "But by the grace of God, I am what I am, and His grace toward me was not in vain." 1 Corinthians 15:10.